ALL YOU NEED
TO KNOW
ABOUT
CLINICAL RESEARCH

ALL YOU NEED
TO KNOW
ABOUT
CLINICAL RESEARCH

A QUICK REFERENCE GUIDE ON CLINICAL RESEARCH

Sanjay Gupta

CR Books

First published in India by
CR Books Pvt. Ltd.
503, Block-C, NDM-2, Netaji Subhash Place, Pitampura, Delhi-110034 (India)
Tel: 011-45121445 Fax : 011-45121435
E-mail : info@crbooks.in, cr.booksltd@gmail.com
Web : www.crbooks.in

First Edition : January 2010
Copyright © CR Books Pvt. Ltd.

The author and publisher have made a conscientious effort to ensure that the
information contained in this book is accurate and in accordance with the
accepted standards at the time of publication. However, in this
rapidly changing world guidelines and practices are subject
to change without prior notification, therefore readers are
advised to confirm these as and when needed.

Typeset in Platino Linotype by Elite Printer
eliteprinter@yahoo.in

Printed and bound by Elite Printer

ISBN 81-908277-1-5

Contents

Preface

Clinical Research is an indispensable part of drug discovery process to ensure that the drug, which is to be marketed, is safe and effective. It is the most expensive and time-consuming component of the drug development process. Since it is a highly specialized job function, it requires specific skill-sets to carry out various operations. Specific skills involves knowledge about clinical trial processes and standards, clinical trial terminologies and abbreviations, essential clinical trial documents, regulatory framework etc. As there are multiple sources of information, it becomes practically impossible to keep them handy for a ready reference.

This book provides a comprehensive understanding of the essential clinical trial elements in a very concise fashion. It is intended to serve as a quick reference guide to all the personnel involved in the conduct of clinical trials as well as to those who plan to enter this field.

I hope the book would leave the desired impression and look forward to receive the feedback from the readers at sanjay@catalystclinicalservices.com

12th January 2010   Sanjay Gupta

Fundamentals of Clinical Research

According to ICH-GCP Guidelines, Clinical Research is any investigation in human subjects intended to discover or verify the clinical, pharmacological and/or other pharmacodynamic effects of an investigational product(s), and/or to identify any adverse reactions to an investigational product(s), and/or to study absorption, distribution, metabolism, and excretion of an investigational product(s) with the object of ascertaining its safety and/or efficacy.

Clinical Research is an indispensable part of drug discovery process to ensure that the drug, which is to be marketed, is safe and effective. It is the most expensive and time-consuming component of the drug development process.

Phases of Clinical Research

Clinical Research is conducted in four phases (I, II, III, and IV) each designed to address different questions. The knowledge gained from one phase is assessed before progressing to the next phase. However, research in a particular phase may continue after the drug has progressed to further stages of development. Based upon data gathered from the pre-clinical (animal testing) trials, the sponsor has some estimation of:

- The drug's therapeutic effect and dose levels
- Toxicity profile and dose levels.

This information is used in the design of Phase I trials.

Phase-I Clinical Trials

These are conducted to establish initial safety, maximum tolerance and pharmacokinetics of a new drug in 20-80 healthy human volunteers.

Phase-I trial addresses:

- How rapidly the drug is absorbed?
- Where is the drug distributed in the body?
- Which organ systems are involved in metabolism of the drug?
- How quickly is the drug eliminated from the body?

During Phase-I trials, sufficient information about the drug's pharmacokinetics and pharmacological effects is obtained to plan a well-controlled Phase-II trial.

Phase-II Clinical Trials

These are conducted for evaluating the efficacy and safety of a new drug. Careful observations are made to determine the dose and adverse reactions in 100-200 patients with the relevant indication. Phase-II trial addresses:

- What is the minimum effective dose?
- What is the maximum tolerated effective dose?
- Is the drug effective in mild, moderate, and severe cases of the disease or condition?
- Is the drug effective for all expected indications?

If a new drug is found to be effective and safe in Phase-II trials, it's development is moved to next phase of development. In case of lack of efficacy the development of drug is stopped at this phase itself.

Phase-III Clinical Trials

These are large, multi-centric trials to establish the safety and efficacy of a new drug *vis-à-vis* existing standard of care/placebo to form the basis for regulatory submission. Phase-III trial addresses:

- Overa'. benefit-risk relationship
- Adv .rse reactions in a large group of patients over a longer period of exposure
- Th . ideal dosage regimen
- Should the drug is allowed to be marketed?

If a new drug is found to be safe and effective in Phase-III trials, a New Drug Application (NDA) is filed to regulatory authorities for seeking marketing permission.

Phase-IV Clinical Trials

These are post marketing studies that are conducted for generating additional safety data on a drug once it is marketed. Phase-IV trial addresses:

- More about the side effects and safety of the drug
- What the long term risks and benefits of the drug are?
- How well the drug works when it's used more widely than in clinical trials?

Regulatory authorities can withdraw the marketing authorization of a drug anytime if there are safety concerns on its usage.

Standards Governing Clinical Research

Declaration of Helsinki, 1964

The World Medial Association (WMA) has developed the Declaration of Helsinki as a statement of ethical principles to provide guidance to physicians and other participants in medical research involving human subjects. Medical research involving human subjects includes research on identifiable human material or identifiable data.

Declaration of Helsinki laid down the Ethical Principles for Medical Research Involving Human Subject and is a major landmark in the evolution of Good Clinical Practices (GCPs).

The Belmont Report, 1979

The Belmont Report is a report created by the former United States Department of Health, Education, and Welfare entitled "Ethical Principles and Guidelines for the Protection of

Human Subjects of Research" and is an important historical document in the field of medical ethics. The report was created on April 18, 1979 and gets its name from the Belmont Conference Center where the document was drafted.

The Belmont Report explains the unifying ethical principles that form the basis for the National Commission's topic-specific reports and the regulations that incorporate its recommendations. The three fundamental ethical principles for using any human subjects for research are:

1. Respect for persons: protecting the autonomy of all people and treating them with courtesy and respect and allowing for informed consent;

2. Beneficence: maximizing benefits for the research project while minimizing risks to the research subjects; and

3. Justice: ensuring reasonable, non-exploitative, and well-considered procedures are administered fairly (the fair distribution of costs and benefits to potential research participants).

ICH - Good Clinical Practice (GCP), 1997

The Food and Drug Administration (FDA) has published a guideline entitled "Good Clinical Practice: Consolidated Guideline". The guideline was prepared under the auspices of the International Conference on Harmonization of Technical Requirements for Registration of Pharmaceuticals for Human Use (ICH). The guideline is intended to define "Good Clinical Practice" and to provide a unified ethical and scientific quality standard for designing, conducting, recording and reporting trials that involve the participation of human subjects. Compliance with this standard provides public assurance that the rights, safety and well being of trial subjects are protected; consistent with the principles that have their origin in the Declaration of Helsinki, and that the clinical trial data are credible.

The objective of the ICH-GCP Guidelines is to provide a unified standard for the European Union (EU), Japan and the United States to facilitate the mutual acceptance of clinical data by the regulatory authorities in these jurisdictions.

The guideline was developed with consideration of the current good clinical practices of the European Union, Japan, and the United States, as well as those of Australia, Canada, the Nordic countries and the World Health Organization (WHO).

The Principles of GCP

1. Clinical trials should be conducted in accordance with the ethical principles that have their origin in the Declaration of Helsinki, and that are consistent with GCP and the applicable regulatory requirement(s).

2. Before a trial is initiated, foreseeable risks and inconveniencies should be weighed against the anticipated benefit for the individual trial subject and society. A trial should be initiated and continued only if the anticipated benefits justify the risks.

3. The rights, safety, and well being of the trial subjects are the most important considerations and should prevail over interests of science and society.

4. The available non-clinical and clinical information on an investigational product should be adequate to support the proposed clinical trial.

5. Clinical trials should be scientifically sound, and describes in a clear, detailed protocol.

6. A trial should be conducted in compliance with the protocol that has received prior institutional review board (IRB)/independent ethics committee (IEC) approval/favorable opinion.

7. The medical care given to, and medical decisions made on behalf of, subjects should always be the responsibility of a qualified physician or, when appropriate, of a qualified dentist.

8. Each individual involved in conducting a trial should be qualified by education, training, and experience to perform his or her respective task(s).

9. Freely given informed consent should be obtained from every subject prior to clinical trial participation.

10. All clinical trial information should be recorded, handled, and stored in a way that allows its accurate reporting, interpretation, and verification.

11. The confidentiality of records that could identify subjects should be protected, respecting the privacy and confidentiality rules in accordance with the applicable regulatory requirement(s).

12. Investigational products should be manufactured, handled, and stored in accordance with applicable good manufacturing practice (GMP). They should be used in accordance with the approved protocol. Systems with procedures that assure the quality of every aspect of the trial should be implemented.

Glossary
of
Clinical Trials
Terminology

A

1. **Abbreviated NDA**
    A type of regulatory application to obtain approval for marketing a generic drug product.

2. **Abstract**
    A brief summary including the objectives, methods, results and conclusion of a clinical trial or any other research work.

3. **Abuse**
    An act that causes physical, social or mental harm or discomfort.

4. **Accelerated Approval**
    A mechanism for speeding the development of drugs that promises significant benefit over existing therapy for serious or life-threatening illnesses where no therapy exists.

5. **Accelerated Development**
    Same as Accelerated Approval.

6. **Accelerated Stability Data**
    Stability data of a drug product under accelerated storage condition as specified by the regulatory guidelines.

7. **Acceptance Letter**
    A letter issued by a clinical trial investigator documenting his/her willingness to participate in a clinical trial and ensuring adherence to the protocol and applicable regulatory guidelines.

8. **Access Control**
    A mechanism by which the access to a clinical trial facility or documents is restricted to authorized individuals only.

9. **Accessibility of Services**
    Same as Access Control.

10. **Accountability**
    Refer to the process, documents and records to demonstrate that investigational product(s) have been used in compliance with protocol and an audit trail is available for all the transactions (receipt, dispensing and return) at any given time point.

11. **Accreditation**
    Evaluation of policies, working procedures and performance of an organization by an accrediting body to ensure that it meets the standards laid down by accrediting body.

12. **Act/Law**
    Refer to legislation.

13. **Action Letter**
    An official communication from regulatory bodies to trial sponsor(s) or investigator(s) or ethics committee(s) documenting its decision.

14. **Active Control**
    A trial design in which subjects are randomly assigned to receive either the standard treatment or the investigational drug.

15. **Active Ingredient**
    The entity (molecule or ion) responsible for the pharmacological action of a drug substance.

16. **Active Moiety**
    Same as Active Ingredient.

17. **Active Treatment Concurrent Control**
    Same as Active Control.

18. **Active Treatment Control**
    Same as Active Control.

19. **Acute Toxicity**
    A type of toxicological testing (usually of 2 weeks) of a drug in 3-4 species of animals for determining its maximum tolerated dose.

20. **Adaptive Designs**
    Refer to a randomization scheme that changes over time depending on the data generated in a trial. In this design the chance of being randomized to one or other of the available treatments at any given point depends on the magnitude of the treatment difference in the data collected so far. The ethical advantage of this scheme is to progressively increase the chance of patients being randomized to the treatment that is performing the best, while decreasing the chance of being randomized to the treatment that is performing the worst.

21. **Addendum**
    A written formal clarification in an essential trial document (such as protocol, informed consent form, investigator's brochure *etc.*)

22. **Adequate and Well Controlled Trial**
    Refer to Phase-3 trials that provide substantial evidence of safety and efficacy of an investigational product which in turn form the basis for its registration.

23. **Adjuvant Therapy**
    Refer to a therapy provided to the patients in order to prevent the disease recurrence after the primary therapy has shown a complete response.

24. **Administrative Expenses**
    Expenses required for meeting the operational and infrastructural requirements of a trial such as telephone, fax, photocopy, travel *etc.*

25. **Admission Criteria**
Refer to the inclusion and exclusion criteria(s) of a trial.

26. **Adverse Drug Event**
Refer to all noxious and unintended responses to a medicinal product at any dose.

27. **Adverse Drug Reaction (ADR)**
Same as adverse drug event.

28. **Adverse Event (AE)**
Any untoward medical occurrence in a patient or clinical investigation subject administered a pharmaceutical product and which does not necessarily have a causal relationship with the treatment.

29. **Adverse Experience**
Any untoward medical occurrence in a patient or clinical investigation subject administered a pharmaceutical product and which does not necessarily have a causal relationship with the treatment.

30. **Advertisement**
A document used for subject recruitment that contains non-coercive trial information and is approved by the institutional ethics committee.

31. **Advocacy and Support Groups**
Organizations and groups that actively support research participants and their families with valuable resources, including self-empowerment and survival tools.

32. **Affirmation Statement**
A statement signed by investigator(s) at the end of trial to document their compliance with ICH-GCP and applicable regulatory requirements.

33. **Agenda**
Refer to a list of topics to be discussed in a meeting.

34. **Agreement**
Refer to a document signed between two or more parties describing the terms of agreement.

35. **Aim of a Study**
Refer to the objective for which a clinical trial is conducted.

36. **Algorithm**
A step-by-step procedure for making a series of choices among alternative decisions to reach an outcome.

37. **Aliquot**
A part that is a definite fraction of a whole sample for laboratory testing or analysis.

38. **Alpha Error (Type-1 Error)**
A type of statistical error. The probability of a Type-1 error (also called the significance level or alpha level) is the probability that the trial will indicate that a therapy is

efficacious (assuming it is not efficacious).

39. **Alternative Hypothesis**
Refer to the study hypothesis that one wishes to investigate and is denoted as H_1 as a standard statistical practice.

40. **Ambulatory Care**
Refer to health services offered on an out-patient basis that does not require hospitalization.

41. **Amendment**
Changes made to essential trial documents (such as protocol, ICD, IB *etc.*) that have an impact on the overall conduct of the study.

42. **Analyte**
A component or a substance that is analyzed employing the analytical techniques.

43. **Ancillary Data**
Data which is not collected on the case report form (*e.g.* ECG interpretations, voice response system data *etc.*).

44. **Ancillary Services**
Refer to diagnostics, laboratory, pharmacy or other services offered by a hospital.

45. **Annotated CRF**
A case report form that has variable and data set names written on it to show where the data can be found in the clinical database.

46. **Annual Reports**
Yearly summary reports submitted to ethics committee or regulatory agencies on the progress of a trial.

47. **Annual Review**
Yearly review of the progress of a trial by ethics committee(s) or regulatory agencies.

48. **Anonymity**
Refer to the de-identified information of a trial participant that in no way can disclose his/her identity.

49. **Applicable Regulatory Requirement(s)**
Any law(s) or regulation(s) addressing the conduct of clinical trials in a country.

50. **Applicant**
A person who submits a trial application to a regulatory agency.

51. **Application**
A trial application submitted by the applicant.

52. **Approvable Letter**
Refer to the action letter from the regulatory agency after the review of a new drug application, which signals that the drug can be approved. It lists minor deficiencies that

can be corrected (often involves labeling change) and possibly requests commitment to do post-approval studies.

53. **Approval**
A letter issued by the ethics committee(s) or regulatory agency (ies) granting the approval to conduct a clinical trial.

54. **Approval Letter**
Refer to the action letter from the regulatory agency after the review of a new drug application, which states that the drug is approved.

55. **Approved Drugs**
All those drugs that are approved by a regulatory authority to be marketed in a country for a particular indication.

56. **Archival**
Refer to the storage of data/records at the end of a clinical trial for the stipulated timeframe.

57. **Archive**
Same as Archival.

58. **Archive Location**
The place or location where the data/records of a trial are stored after the completion of a trial.

59. **Arm**
Refer to a treatment group in a randomized trial.

60. **Assent**
A process by which a child voluntarily confirms his or her willingness to participate in a clinical trial after having been informed of all the aspects of the trial that is relevant to his/her decision to participate.

61. **Assurance**
A formal written, binding commitment submitted to regulatory authorities by trial investigator(s) and sponsor(s) assuring their compliance with all applicable regulatory requirements.

62. **As-treated**
A statistical approach in which patients are analyzed according to the treatment that they actually received, rather than the one to which they were randomized. The goal of an as-treated analysis is often to assess the true biological effects of therapy rather than the combination of biological effects and compliance to treatment. However, the limitation of this approach is that the balance provided by randomization is potentially lost.

63. **Attribution**
Investigator's assessment on the relatedness of an adverse event to the investigational product.

64. **Audit**
A systematic and independent examination of trial related activities and documents to determine whether the evaluated trial related activities were conducted, and the data were recorded, analyzed and accurately reported according to the protocol, sponsor's Standard Operating Procedures (SOPs), Good Clinical Practice (GCP), and the applicable regulatory requirement(s).

65. **Audit Certificate**
Document that certifies that an audit has taken place.

66. **Audit Finding(s)**
A written conclusion of the audit results by the auditor.

67. **Audit Report**
A written evaluation of the audit results by the auditor.

68. **Audit Trail**
Refer to the documentation of activities that allows reconstruction of the course of events.

69. **Authorization**
Permission to use and share a subject's protected health information for the purposes of the research study.

70. **Authorized Personnel**
A personnel who has the authority to access and review the trial related documents and activities.

71. **Autonomy**
Refer to the personal capacity to make choices, consider alternatives and act without undue influence or interference of others.

72. **Autopsy**
Dissection of a dead body to determine the cause of death and relevant medical facts.

3

B

73. **Back Translation**
Refer to a process by which vernacular language translation of a trial document is back translated in to English.

74. **Back-up**
Refer to the process of making a copy of important data onto a different storage medium.

75. **Balanced Study**
A study in which a particular type of subject is equally represented in each study group.

76. **Bar Charts**
Refer to a type of statistical chart that displays the distribution of levels (percentages or count) of a categorical variable.

77. **Bar Code**
A pattern of black vertical lines containing the coded information to uniquely identify and/or track clinical supplies.

78. **Baseline**
Refer to the pre-treatment time-point of a clinical trial.

79. **Baseline Assessment**
Refer to the pre-treatment evaluations on study subjects as they enter a clinical trial and before any investigational product or interventions are given.

80. **Belmont Report**
A document that is part of the Federal Register and sets forth the foundation of rules for all government funded research involving human subjects. The three basic ethical principles as stated in Belmont report include: (1) respect for persons (2) beneficence, and (3) justice.

81. **Benefit**
Refer to the achievement of a desired outcome in a clinical trial.

82. **Benefit Risk Assessment**
Refer to the evaluation of risks that a clinical trial poses to the study subjects *vis-à-vis* its benefits.

83. **Beta Error**
A type of statistical error. The probability of a Type-2 error (also called the beta level) is the probability that the trial will fail to show that a therapy is efficacious (assuming it is efficacious).

84. **Bias**
Refer to a systematic tendency built into the design or conduct of the study, which skews the results. Bias can occur systematically across all treatment groups leading to an under or over estimation of the results.

85. **Bidding**
A process of submitting competitive proposals to a trial sponsor (containing costs, timelines, deliverables *etc.*) by different individuals/organizations.

86. **Bioanalytical Assays**
Refer to the methods for quantitative measurement of a drug, metabolites or chemicals in biological fluids.

87. **Bioavailability**
Refer to the amount of drug that is absorbed after administration by route X compared with the amount of drug that is absorbed after intravenous (I.V.) administration where X is any route of drug administration other than I.V.

88. **Bioavailability Studies**
Studies carried out to assess and compare the pharmacokinetic parameters of a test product (usually a generic version) compared to a reference drug (usually the innovator drug).

89. **Bioinformatics**
Refer to information systems developed for analysis of biological data (particularly genomic data). It is used for gene identification and mapping.

90. **Biologic**
Any therapeutic serum, toxin, anti-toxin, or analogous microbial product used for the prevention, treatment, or cure of diseases or injuries in human.

91. **Biological Marker**
Refer to a biological molecule used as a marker to measure the progress of a disease or effects of a treatment.

92. **Biological Product**
Same as Biologic.

93. **Biological Safety Officer**
Personnel having the capabilities of evaluating and monitoring the safety of biological products.

94. **Biometric Identifier**
Individual identifier based on physical characteristic such as a fingerprint, thumb impression, retina scan *etc.*

95. **Biometrics**
Measurable physical characteristic or personal behavioral trait used to recognize or verify the identity of an individual.

96. **Biopharmaceutics**
Refer to the study of the relationship between physical and chemical properties, dosage and administration of a drug and its activity in humans and animals.

97. **Biostatistics**
Refer to the application of statistics to medicine which is a process of collecting, recording and summarizing data from experiments, records and surveys.

98. **Biotechnology**
Refer to any technique that uses living organisms, or substances from organisms, biological systems, or processes to make or modify a product or process, to change plants or animals, or to develop micro-organisms for specific uses.

99. **Blinded Medications**
Refer to investigational products that appear identical in size, shape, color and all other attributes so that the patients and/or investigator remains unaware of the type of treatment being administered.

100. **Blinded Study Design**
Clinical study designs in which one or more parties to the trial are kept unaware of the treatment assignment(s). These study designs reduces bias by preserving symmetry in the observer's measurements and assessments.

101. **Blinded Trials**
Same as Blinded Study Design.

102. **Blinding**
A procedure in which one or more parties to the trial are kept unaware of the treatment assignment(s). Single-blinding usually refers to the subject(s) being unaware, and double blinding usually refers to the subject(s), investigator(s), monitor, and, in some cases, data analyst(s) being unaware of the treatment assignment(s). Blinding reduces bias by preserving symmetry in the observer's measurements and assessments.

103. **Blinding / Masking**
A process in which the clinicians and/or the patients remain unaware of the type of treatment being administered to avoid bias.

104. **Block Size**
Refer to smaller fixed size randomization groups to ensure that an approximately equal number of subjects receive each study treatment even if each participating center does not recruit its full quota of subjects.

105. **Body Surface Area**
Refer to total surface area of the human body which is widely used for the calculation of drug dosages of cancer medicines.

106. **Box Plots**
Refer to a type of statistical chart that displays information about the distribution of a numeric variable. It is useful for displaying the relationship between a numeric variable and a categorical variable.

107. **Breakdown**
Refer to getting out of order.

108. **Budgeting**
An estimate of the total cost involved for a particular activity or for the conduct of entire clinical trial.

109. **Bulk Supplies**
Refer to large stocks of clinical trial supplies.

110. **Business Associate**
A person or organization that uses protected health information (PHI) to perform a function or activity on behalf of a covered entity, but is not part of the covered entity's workforce.

4

C

111. Cache
Refer to storage area on a computer's hard drive where the web pages and/or graphic elements are stored temporarily.

112. Cadaver
The body of a deceased person used for imparting medical education.

113. Cadaveric Transplant
The surgical procedure of excising a kidney from a deceased individual and implanting it into a suitable recipient.

114. Calibration
A quality control process of standardizing the equipments, machines, apparatus *etc.* used in scientific testing.

115. Candidate
A term used for potential drug substance in the drug discovery process.

116. Capacity
The ability to understand the purpose, procedures, risks, benefits and alternatives to a research study, including the ability to express a choice about participation and to understand that a refusal to participate involves no penalty or loss of benefits to which the person is otherwise entitled.

117. Carcinogenic
Refer to potential of a substance to cause cancer.

118. Caregiver
A person who provides social, emotional, medical and financial support to an individual.

119. Carry Over Effect
Effects of treatment that persist after treatment has been stopped.

120. Case Control Study
A type of retrospective study comparing persons with a given condition or disease (the cases) and persons without the condition or disease (the controls) with respect to antecedent factors.

121. Case History Record
A complete record of a patient's disease history entered in hospital files, out-patient charts or medical records.

122. Case Management
A process of providing the health care services to an individual.

123. **Case Report Form (CRF)**
A printed, optical, or electronic document designed to record all of the protocol-required information on each trial subject.

124. **Case Study Form**
Same as Case Report Form.

125. **Catastrophic Illness**
An extremely serious and expensive health problem that could be life threatening or may cause life-long disability.

126. **Categorical Data**
Refer to a type of data, which can be divided into groups for *e.g.* race, sex, age group, educational level *etc.*

127. **Causality**
Determination of the relatedness of an adverse event to the study drug or procedure.

128. **Causality Assessment**
Same as Causality.

129. **Censored Data**
An observation is said to be censored when the event of interest (*e.g.* survival, death, response *etc.*) is not recorded for a particular patient.

130. **Censoring**
An observation is said to be censored when the event of interest is not recorded for a particular patient. For *e.g.* in a study of survival times following a cancer treatment, if few patients are alive at the end of required follow-up period than their survival time will be censored at that time point.

131. **Central Data Coordinating Center**
An organization or department having a centralized function of managing the trial data.

132. **Central Ethics Committee**
An independent body, constituted of medical professionals and non-medical members, whose responsibility is to ensure the protection of the rights, safety and well being of human subjects involved in a clinical trial and to provide public assurance of that protection, by, among other things, reviewing and approving/providing favorable opinion on, the trial protocol, the suitability of the investigator(s), facilities, and the methods and material to be used in obtaining and documenting informed consent of the trial subjects.

133. **Central Institutional Review Board**
Same as Central Ethics Committee.

134. **Central Lab**
A laboratory having a centralized function of evaluating the protocol required lab parameters for all the sites involved in a trial.

135. **Central Review Board**
Same as Central Ethics Committee.

136. **Central Tendency**
Refer to the central value from a series of observation around which all other observations are dispersed. In any large series, nearly 50% observations lie above while the remaining 50% lie below the central value. It indicates the central tendency or concentration of all other observations around the central value.

137. **Certificate of Analysis (COA)**
An analytical report of a batch of investigational product highlighting its content uniformity and percentage purity. COA is generated for each batch of medicinal products.

138. **Certification/Accreditation**
Evaluation of policies, working procedures and performance of an organization by an accrediting body to ensure that it meets the standards laid down by accrediting body.

139. **21 CFR Part 11 Regulations**
Regulations allowing FDA to accept electronic records and signatures in place of paper records and handwritten signatures.

140. **Chi-square Test**
A statistical test to determine whether there is an association between two categorical variables. The relationship between the categorical variables is presented in a table containing r (rows) and c (columns).

141. **Chronic Toxicity**
A type of toxicological testing (up to 12 months studies) of a drug in rats and a non-rodent species of animals to determine adverse effects with repeated daily dosing.

142. **Circadian Rhythm**
Refer to biological timing and rhythmicity that in human beings is characterized by cycles of approximately 24 hours.

143. **Class 1 Device**
One of 3 classifications of medical devices by the Food and Drug Administration according to its potential risks or hazards. Examples include elastic bandages, exam gloves, and hand-held surgical instruments.

144. **Class 2 Device**
One of 3 classifications of medical devices by the Food and Drug Administration according to its potential risks or hazards. Examples include powered wheel chairs, infusion pumps, and surgical drapes.

145. **Class 3 Device**
One of 3 classifications of medical devices by the Food and Drug Administration according to its potential risks or hazards. Examples include replacement heart valves, silicone gel-filled breast implants.

146. **Class Codes**
Codes used by the Food and Drug Administration to classify medical devices according to the potential risks or hazards.

147. **Clean Database**
A clinical trial database in which all the validation queries have been resolved and which is ready for the analysis.

148. **Client**
Refer to a program (the client) that makes a service request of another program (the server).

149. **Clinical**
Related to human participants.

150. **Clinical Coordinator**
A person who assist the investigator in the management of a trial at a site.

151. **Clinical Data Interchange Standards Consortium (CDISC)**
An organization whose mission is "to develop and support global, platform-independent data standards that enable information system interoperability to improve medical research and related areas of healthcare".

152. **Clinical Data Management**
The process of managing the trial data right from the development of case report form to the collection, entry, validation, query resolution and statistical analysis.

153. **Clinical Development Plan**
A written document containing the clinical strategy for the development of an investigational product.

154. **Clinical Efficacy**
A product's ability to produce beneficial effects on the course of a disease.

155. **Clinical Equipoise**
Refer to ethical principle of assigning patients to different treatment arms, where the clinician does not have preference of any arm over the others. In this approach every subject has an equal chance of getting randomized to any of the treatment arm.

156. **Clinical Hold**
A decision of the Food and Drug Administration to put the clinical development of a drug on hold when it cannot confirm that the study can be conducted without unreasonable risk to the subject.

157. **Clinical Investigator**
A person responsible for the conduct of the clinical trial at a trial site. If a trial is conducted by a team of individuals at a trial site, the investigator is the responsible leader of the team and may be called the principal investigator.

158. **Clinical Laboratory Improvement Amendments**
United States law passed in 1988 that established quality standards for laboratories

testing to ensure the accuracy, reliability and timeliness of test results regardless of where the test was performed.

159. **Clinical Observations**
A note or a record of clinical sign and symptoms of a patient.

160. **Clinical Performance Measure**
A method to estimate or monitor the extent to which the actions of a health care provider conforms to the practice guidelines, medical review criteria, or standards of quality.

161. **Clinical Pharmacology**
The science of drugs and their clinical use.

162. **Clinical Phase**
The time period between the initiation and completion of a trial at a site.

163. **Clinical Research and Development**
An organized research conducted on human beings to investigate the safety and efficacy of a drug.

164. **Clinical Research Assistant**
A person employed by the sponsor, or contract research organization acting on behalf of a sponsor, who assist in overall trial management and ensures compliance with applicable regulatory guidelines.

165. **Clinical Research Associate**
A person employed by a sponsor, or contract research organization acting on behalf of a sponsor, who monitors the conduct as well as progress of a trial at investigator sites participating in the trial.

166. **Clinical Research Center**
A dedicated area at a trial site for the conduct of clinical trials.

167. **Clinical Research Coordinator (CRC)**
A person employed at clinical investigator's site to record the clinical trial data in compliance with protocol, GCP and applicable regulatory guidelines. The investigator delegates specific duties to CRC. CRC may also be called as research/study/healthcare coordinator, research nurse or protocol nurse.

168. **Clinical Significance**
Changes in a subject's clinical condition considered as important and which may or may not be related to the study drug(s).

169. **Clinical Study**
Any investigation in human subjects intended to discover or verify the clinical, pharmacological, and/or other pharmacodynamic effects of an investigational product(s), and/or to identify any adverse reactions, and/or to study absorption, distribution, metabolism, and excretion of an investigational product(s) with the object of ascertaining its safety and efficacy.

170. Clinical Study Agreement

A document signed and dated by the investigator and the sponsor of a trial that describes the responsibility, timelines, payment schedule and other relevant terms of agreement between the involved parties.

171. Clinical Study Materials

Study supplies (such as study test article, laboratory supplies, case report forms *etc.*) provided by the sponsor to the investigator.

172. Clinical Study Report

Written description of the outcome of a trial enumerating the clinical and statistical interpretations.

173. Clinical Testing

Testing in human beings.

174. Clinical Trial

Any investigation in human subjects intended to discover or verify the clinical, pharmacological, and/or other pharmacodynamic effects of an investigational product(s), and/or to identify any adverse reactions, and/or to study absorption, distribution, metabolism, and excretion of an investigational product(s) with the object of ascertaining its safety and efficacy.

175. Clinical Trial Agreement

A document signed and dated by the investigator and the sponsor of a trial that describes the responsibility, timelines, payment schedule and other relevant terms of agreement between the involved parties.

176. Clinical Trial Coordinator

A person employed at clinical investigator's site to record the clinical trial data in compliance with protocol, GCP and applicable regulatory guidelines. The investigator delegates specific duties to CRC. CRC may also be called as research/study/healthcare coordinator, research nurse or protocol nurse.

177. Clinical Trial Exemption

Refer to the formal submission of a trial application (including preclinical, pharmacology, safety, manufacturing and clinical data) by a Sponsor to the Regulatory Agency followed by obtaining no objection for initiating the trial.

178. Clinical Trial Material Destruction Certificate

A certificate to document the destruction of used and unused clinical trial material (*e.g.* investigational medicinal product, lab kits, documents *etc.*) for the purpose of accountability and ensuring compliance with applicable regulations.

179. Clinical Trial Materials

Complete set of supplies (*e.g.* documents, laboratory, and investigational medicinal product *etc.*) provided to an investigator.

180. Clinical Trial Material Label

Label affixed to investigational product containing essential information on the product and the manufacturer.

181. **Clinical Trial Monitoring**
The act of overseeing the progress of a clinical trial, and of ensuring that it is conducted, recorded, and reported in accordance with the Protocol, Standard Operating Procedures (SOPs), Good Clinical Practice (GCP), and the applicable regulatory requirements. Clinical trial monitoring is usually performed by a monitor or clinical research associate, appointed by the trial sponsor.

182. **Clinical Trial Office**
A dedicated area for the conduct of clinical trials having required infrastructure and access control.

183. **Clinical Trial Report**
Written description of the outcome of a trial enumerating the clinical and statistical interpretations.

184. **Clinical Trial Simulation**
An effort to devise *in silico* simulations of human physiology and genetic variation to identify compounds that will eventually fail in the drug development process.

185. **Close Relative**
Any person (eighteen years of age or older) who is related to the prospective trial subject and has maintained such regular contact with the subject to be familiar with his or her activities, health, and religious or moral beliefs.

186. **Closed System**
An environment in which system access is controlled by persons who are responsible for the content of electronic records that is on the system.

187. **Code of Federal Regulations (CFR)**
An annual codification of the general and permanent rules published in the Federal Register (U.S) by the executive departments and agencies of the Federal Government. The CFR is divided into 50 titles representing broad areas of Federal regulation. Each Title is divided into chapters that are assigned to agencies issuing regulations pertaining to that broad subject area. Each chapter is divided into parts and each part is then divided into sections, the basic unit of the CFR.

188. **Coding**
The process of assigning data/supplies to categories having a unique identifier.

189. **Coercion**
Refer to unacceptable subject recruitment procedures, which involves undue inducement, duress or indirect pressure to participate in a clinical trial.

190. **Co-factor Data**
Data on important co-factors associated with a disease state. For *e.g.* demographic data, performance status, prior treatments, stage of disease, laboratory parameters *etc.*

191. **Cognitive Impairment**
Refer to a medical condition in which an individual's capacity for judgment and reasoning is significantly diminished.

192. **Cognitively Impaired**
Same as Cognitive Impairment.

193. **Cohort**
A group of individuals identified on the basis of a common experience or characteristic that is usually monitored over time from the point of assembly. For *e.g.* comparing the response of treatment in males *vs.* females; elderly *vs.* young patients *etc.*

194. **Cohort Study**
Longitudinal studies in which the sample is a cohort. It could be a prospective study such as follow-up of morbidity and mortality in infants from birth to one year of age or retrospective study such as number of persons in the same population who suffered from polio in last 2 years.

195. **Co-investigator**
An individual who shares study responsibilities with the investigator at a trial site.

196. **Combinatorial Biosynthesis**
A technique for modeling and building libraries of chemical compounds for consideration as drug candidates.

197. **Combinatorial Chemistry**
A technique of modifying an existing compound chemically to act on a selected target.

198. **Commercial IND**
A type of Investigational New Drug Application that is submitted by companies whose ultimate goal is to obtain marketing approval of a new product.

199. **Common Rule**
United States agreement to cover all Federal-sponsored research by a common set of regulations.

200. **Common Technical Document (CTD)**
An ICH defined format for a regulatory submission that is considered acceptable in Japan, Europe, the United States and Canada.

201. **Communications**
Documents narrating the conversation or discussion between two or more parties for *e.g.* letters, e-mails, fax, telephonic logs *etc.*

202. **Comparative Study**
A clinical trial design in which investigational product is compared with an approved drug or placebo.

203. **Comparator**
A marketed product (*i.e.*, active control), or placebo, used as a reference in a clinical trial.

204. **Comparison Group**
A group of trial participants having similar characteristics in terms of age, gender, race *etc*.

205. **Comparison Tests**
Statistical tests used for drawing conclusions about differences between two or more groups.

206. **Compassionate Use**
A method of providing experimental drugs/therapeutics prior to their final regulatory approval for use in humans. This procedure is applicable for very sick individuals who does not have any other treatment options for their medical management. "Compassionate Use" requires a case-to-case approval from the regulatory authorities.

207. **Compensation**
Refer to medical care or payment provided to a subject for trial related injuries.

208. **Competence**
Ability to act on one's own behalf after having understood all the consequences thereon.

209. **Competent Authority**
Authorities that grants trial permission and monitors compliance with applicable regulatory guidelines.

210. **Complementary Medicine**
An alternate system of medicine based on different principles than allopathic system.

211. **Compliance**
Adherence to study protocol, Good Clinical Practice (GCP) guidelines, and the applicable regulatory requirements.

212. **Computer Validation**
The process of evaluation of the hardware and software of a system to ensure accurate and reliable compliance with user requirements.

213. **Concomitant Medication**
Medication taken by a study subject for diseases/medical conditions other than the study disease.

214. **Concurrent Standard Therapy**
Standard treatment that a subject receives while participating in a clinical trial which is not the treatment under investigation. For *e.g.* in a trial of chemotherapy induced anemia, chemotherapy is concurrent standard therapy while treatment for anemia is the treatment under investigation.

215. **Concurrently**
In parallel or simultaneously.

216. **Confidence Intervals**
It represents a plausible range for the population value results from the sample. 95%

confidence interval is used most frequently in statistical analysis which corresponds to a p-value of less than 0.05.

217. Confidentiality
Prevention of disclosure of proprietary information to unauthorized individuals.

218. Confidentiality Statement
Statement included in the informed consent form that states 'identification of a subject will be kept confidential and to the extent permitted by applicable laws and regulations will not be made publicly available'.

219. Conflict of Interest
Refer to professional, personal or financial interest that can unduly bias an individual to perform his/her duties.

220. Conformity Assessment
A process by which compliance with essential requirement is evaluated.

221. Confounding
A type of bias that occurs when the two treatment groups being compared contains different type of patients. When this happens, it is not possible to identify whether any observed differences between the treatments have arisen from inherent differences between the treatments or between the patients being compared.

222. Consent
A process by which a subject voluntarily confirms his or her willingness to participate in a particular trial, after having been informed of all aspects of the trial that are relevant to the subject's decision to participate. Informed consent is documented by means of a written, signed, and dated informed consent form.

223. Consent Form
Document used to obtain the written, signed and dated consent from a subject for the voluntary participation in a trial.

224. Consortium
An agreement between a university and corporate partners for a specific research project or program.

225. Consultant
An independent personnel or organization hired for performing a specific duty.

226. Consulting Agreement
Document used to enlist the responsibilities and obligations of a consultant.

227. Continuing Medical Education
An ongoing process of learning new advancements and researches that has taken place in medical science.

228. Continuing Review
Periodic review by Ethics Committee for the purpose of re-approving, disapproving,

terminating or suspending an already approved study.

229. **Continuous Quality Improvement**
An ongoing process of improving the quality via quality improvement programs.

230. **Contract**
A written, dated, and signed agreement between two or more involved parties that sets out arrangements on delegation and distribution of tasks and obligations and, if appropriate, on financial matters. The protocol may serve as the basis of a contract. It may also be called as Letter of Agreement (LOA) or Professional Services Agreement (PSA).

231. **Contract Research Organization (CRO)**
A person or an organization (commercial, academic, or other) contracted by the sponsor to perform one or more of a sponsor's trial-related duties and functions.

232. **Contraindication**
A condition in which a drug/medication should not be administered.

233. **Control Group**
Refer to a comparison group of study subjects in a trial who are not treated with the investigational agent. The subjects in this group may receive no therapy, a different therapy, or a placebo.

234. **Controlled Comparisons**
Clinical trial designs to ensure the efficacy assessment of a new treatment against a meaningful comparator. It is appropriate to compare a new treatment or strategy against the current standard of care or a placebo if no standard of care exists.

235. **Controlled Study**
A clinical study that contains a control group (who receives no therapy, a different therapy or a placebo) for the overall safety and efficacy comparison of the investigational agent.

236. **Coordinating Center**
An organization or part of an organization with a centralized function of managing a clinical study (*e.g.* data management, monitoring, supplies management *etc.*) in a multicentric trial.

237. **Coordinating Committee**
A committee that a sponsor may organize to coordinate the conduct of a multicentric trial.

238. **Coordinating Investigator**
An investigator responsible for the coordination of investigators at different centers participating in a multicentric trial.

239. **Co-Principal Investigator**
An individual who shares the clinical trial responsibility with principal investigator.

240. **Copyright**
A law which excludes the users (for a limited period of time) from using original works of authorship fixed in any tangible medium of expression.

241. **Correlation**
A measure of the strength of the relationship between two variables *e.g.* the positive correlation between cigarette smoking and the incidence of lung cancer; the negative correlation between age and normal vision.

242. **Correlation Coefficient**
A measure that determines the degree to which the movement of two variables is associated.

243. **Correspondence**
Documents narrating the conversation or discussion between two or more parties for *e.g.* letters, e-mails, fax, telephonic logs *etc.*

244. **Cost Benefit Analysis**
Analysis to quantify the benefits associated with the use of a particular medication *vis-à-vis* direct cost implications.

245. **Cost Effectiveness Analysis**
Analysis to quantify the effectiveness or outcome (*e.g.* overall survival) associated with the use of a particular medication *vis-à-vis* direct cost implications.

246. **Cost Estimate**
An estimate of the total cost implication for carrying out a particular activity.

247. **Covered Clinical Study**
Studies that aim to establish the efficacy of the product.

248. **Covariate**
Refer to a variable that has an influence on another dependent variable. For *e.g.* advance stage disease may be a covariate for mortality rate in a clinical trial.

249. **Covered Entity**
Refer to three types of entities that must comply with the Health Insurance Portability and Accountability Act (HIPAA) Privacy Rule. These include health care providers, health plans and health care clearinghouses.

250. **Covered Functions**
Functions carried out by covered entity.

251. **Covered Transaction**
Transactions carried out by covered entity.

252. **Cox-proportional Hazard Models**
Statistical models to test the significance and relative importance of the co-factors,

which influence the survival experiences in different groups.

253. **Crossover**
A strategy employed in clinical trials comparing two treatments, where each patient receives both the treatments, one followed by the other, and the treatments are compared on the basis of within patient comparisons.

254. **Crossover Design**
A strategy employed in clinical trials comparing two treatments, where each patient receives both the treatments, one followed by the other, and the treatments are compared on the basis of within patient comparisons.

255. **Crossover Studies**
Same as Crossover Design.

256. **Clinical Trial Notification Scheme (CTN)**
Under this scheme, the sponsor of a clinical trial is required to obtain approval for their study from an Institutional Ethics Committee, after which they simply notify to the regulatory agency and can commence the study.

257. **Clinical Trial Exemption Scheme (CTX)**
This scheme requires a formal submission of clinical trial application to be reviewed and approved by the regulatory authority.

258. **Curriculum Vitae (CV)**
Document containing the details on the qualification, experience and personal information of a person.

259. **Custodial Care**
Non-skilled personal care such as help with activities of daily living like bathing, dressing, eating, getting in or out of a bed or chair and using the bathroom.

5

D

260. **Data**
Refer to recorded information regardless of form (manual or electronic).

261. **Data and Safety Monitoring Board**
Independent data monitoring committee that may be established by the sponsor to periodically assess the progress of a clinical trial, the safety data, the critical efficacy endpoints and to recommend to the sponsor whether to continue, modify or stop a trial.

262. **Data Archival**
The storage of data under proper environmental and access control after the completion of trial.

263. **Data Audit Trail**
The documentation that tracks the changes that have been made to the recorded data and/or databases.

264. **Data Clarification Form**
A document generated to resolve query on a particular page of case report form after the same has been collected from the site.

265. **Data Collection**
Collection of information about each subject during the course of a trial.

266. **Data Collection Form**
A document designed to record the protocol required information on each trial subject. It can be either in a printed or an electronic format.

267. **Data Condition**
Description of the circumstances in which a particular data is required.

268. **Data Coordinating Center**
An organization or a department having a centralized data management functions for a multi-centric trial.

269. **Data Dictionary**
A document that characterizes the data content of a system.

270. **Data Element**
Refer to recorded information regardless of form (manual or electronic).

271. **Data Error**
Errors in either collection or recording of clinical trial data.

272. **Data Form**
A printed, optical, or electronic document designed to record all of the protocol required information on each trial subject.

273. **Data Integrity**
The accuracy and validity of a given data.

274. **Data Lock**
The process of converting the data entered in an electronic data entry system to 'read only' format so that no further changes can be made to the database. The data at this stage is ready to be processed for statistical analysis.

275. **Data Management**
The process of handling the data (recording, analyzing and reporting) collected during a clinical trial.

276. **Data Management Planning**
A written document to describe the data management strategy to be employed in a clinical trial.

277. **Data Mapping**
The process of matching one set of data elements to their closest equivalents in another data set or in a reference dictionary.

278. **Data Monitoring**
The process of verifying the data entered in the case report form against the source data in order to establish its accuracy and completeness.

279. **Data Monitoring Committee**
Independent data monitoring committee that may be established by the sponsor to periodically assess the progress of a clinical trial, the safety data, the critical efficacy endpoints and to recommend to the sponsor whether to continue, modify or stop a trial.

280. **Data Outputs**
Analytical reports/tables for a given dataset.

281. **Data Point(s)**
Text or numbers generated during the analysis of a clinical trial data.

282. **Data Query**
A query generated during the data entry or review of a clinical trial data.

283. **Data Safety Committee**
An independent committee established by the sponsor to assess at intervals that participants are not exposed to undue risk and to recommend to the sponsor whether to continue, modify or stop a trial.

284. **Data Safety Monitoring Board (DSMB)**
Independent data monitoring committee that may be established by the sponsor to periodically assess the progress of a clinical trial, the safety data, the critical efficacy endpoints and to recommend to the sponsor whether to continue, modify or stop a trial.

285. **Data Validation**
A process of ensuring the accuracy and completeness of a clinical trial data using manual checks, computerized generated edits, reports or listings as defined in the data validation plan.

286. **Data Validation Plan**
Data validation plan documents the methods and strategy used to determine the point at which the overall study data will be considered as validated.

287. **Data Verification**
Process of checking the accuracy of the data that has been entered into a computer database.

288. **Database**
An electronic platform that contains the data generated from a clinical trial.

289. **Data Base Quality Review (DBQR)**
A comparison of case report form and ancillary data to the raw data in the clinical trial reporting database. The purpose of DBQR is to demonstrate the accuracy of the data processing and to ensure that the data received from the investigator site and various laboratories matches the data output from the reporting database.

290. **Death**
A fatal outcome of an adverse event or the primary study disease. In clinical trials death is considered as one of the criteria for qualifying an adverse event as a serious adverse event.

291. **Debarment List**
A list published on US-FDA's website containing the names of personnel that have been disqualified for conducting clinical trials on grounds of serious misconduct or medical fraud.

292. **Deception**
Refer to intentionally misleading or withholding information.

293. **Decisionally Incapacitated Individual**
An individual who is at least 18 years of age, but who cannot give a valid informed consent to participate in a research due to his inability to understand the nature, extent, or consequence of the proposed participation.

294. **Declaration of Helsinki**
A series of guidelines first adopted by the 18th World Medical Assembly in Helsinki, Finland in 1964. The Declaration addresses ethical issues for physicians conducting biomedical research involving human subjects. Recommendations include the procedures required to ensure subject safety in clinical trials, including informed consent and Ethics Committee reviews.

295. **Decoding Procedure**
Refer to a procedure for breaking the treatment codes (unblinding) in a blinded clinical trial.

296. **De-identification**
The process of removal of all the elements that makes data individually identifiable.

297. Delegation
Allocation of specific trial related duties to the individual study team members in a clinical trial.

298. Delegation of Authority Log
A document that enlists the specific trial related duties performed by individual study team members along with their signatures and/or initials.

299. Demographic Data
Refer to the characteristics of study participants (such as gender, age, family medical history, and other characteristics) relevant to the study in which they are enrolled.

300. Dependent Variables
Dependent variables represent the outcomes that are measured in a clinical trial and that are expected to change as a result of an experimental manipulation of the independent variable(s).

301. Descriptive Study
Any study which is not purely an experimental study.

302. Designated Personnel
Personnel that have been assigned specific trial related duties.

303. Destruction Certificate
A document that captures the description and the quantity of a clinical trial material (used or unused) destroyed either during or at the end of the trial.

304. Destruction Records
Same as Destruction Certificate.

305. Deviation
Non-compliance to either protocol schedule of events or standard operating procedures.

306. Deviation File Note
A document that describes a deviation along with root cause and rectification analysis. Deviation file note contains the signature of the personnel who is responsible for the deviation and the personnel who is authorizing the deviation.

307. Device
An instrument, apparatus, implement, machine, contrivance, implant, *in vitro* reagent, or other similar or related article, including any component, part or accessory, which is intended for use in the diagnosis, cure, treatment or prevention of disease.

308. Diagnosis
The determination of the nature of a disease.

309. Diagnosis Code
International classification codes for a particular diagnosis.

310. Diagnostics
Tests used for the diagnosis of a disease.

311. Diary/Cards
Forms containing study specific information (safety, efficacy, drug compliance *etc.*) required to be filled in by the study subjects.

312. Digital Signature
An electronic signature based upon cryptographic methods of originator authentication such that the identity of the signer and the integrity of the data can be verified.

313. Direct Access
An environment in which the access to trial related information is not controlled.

314. Direct Costs
Actual cost associated with an activity.

315. Direct Data Entry
An environment in which trial data is directly entered into a web-based data management system.

316. Directorate General of Foreign Trade (DGFT)
The office of Directorate General of Foreign Trade (DGFT) which was earlier responsible for granting the export license for the shipment of biological specimens out of India.

317. Disability
A substantial disruption of a person's ability to conduct normal life functions.

318. Disclosure
Refer to release of protected health information of a study subject by one entity to another entity.

319. Discovery
A new invention (in relation to drug discovery it refers to the identification and optimization of initial hit compounds or lead molecules).

320. Disease
A condition that impairs the normal functioning of an organism or body.

321. Distribution
Refer to the circulation of drug or its metabolite in the entire body through blood.

322. Documentation
Refer to records that describe or document study methods, conduct and results.

323. Domain Name
Name of a website/web server.

324. Dosage Form
Refer to the pharmaceutical delivery system for a drug product (*e.g.* tablet, capsule, suspension, ointment, injection *etc.*).

325. Dosage Regimen
Refer to the amount of a drug product to be given at each specific dosing time.

326. Dose
The amount of drug to be used for a medical condition.

327. Dose Comparison Control
Refer to subjects who are randomly assigned to at least one of the two doses of study drug.

328. Dose Range Finding Study
A study (clinical trial) to compare two or more doses of the same drug product.

329. Dose Ranging Study
A clinical trial in which two or more doses of an agent (such as a drug) are tested against each other to determine which dose works best and is least harmful.

330. Dosing Schedule
Refer to the amount of a drug product to be given at each specific dosing time.

331. Dossier/Regulatory Dossier
Documents submitted to the regulatory agencies in a pre-specified format for obtaining trial permission.

332. Double Blind
The design of a study in which neither the investigator nor the subject knows which medication (or placebo) the subject is receiving.

333. Double Data Entry
Separate entry of clinical trial data (in a data management system) by two different individuals to minimize the data entry errors.

334. Double Dummy
A technique that enables a trial comparing two different dosage forms (*e.g.* tablets and capsules) to be conducted in a double blind manner. In this design a subject receives both dosage forms at the same time whereby one of the dosage form is a placebo.

335. Double Masked
Same as Double Blind.

336. Drop Out
Refer to a study subject who does not complete the protocol specified visits in a clinical trial.

337. Drug
As defined by the Food, Drug and Cosmetic Act, drugs are 'articles (other than food) intended for the use in the diagnosis, cure, mitigation, treatment, or prevention of disease in man or other animals or to affect the structure or any function of the body of man or other animals.'

338. Drug Accountability
A process by which accountability of each unit of an investigational product is established.

339. **Drug Accountability Logs**
Logs designed to capture all the transactions (such as receipt, dispensing, return, destruction *etc.*) of an investigational product in order to ascertain 100% accountability at any time-point.

340. **Drug/Device Accountability Records (DAR)**
Same as Drug Accountability Logs.

341. **Drug Candidate**
Refer to an 'article' that has a potential to become a successful drug through systematic clinical trial investigations.

342. **Drug Controller General of India (DCGI)**
The office of Drug Controller General of India under Central Drug standard control organization (CDSCO) having the prime responsibility for regulating clinical trials in India.

343. **Drug Development**
Refer to the clinical development of a drug candidate through various phases of clinical trials.

344. **Drug Discovery**
Refer to the pre-clinical development of a drug candidate.

345. **Drug Level**
Refer to the amount of drug (investigational product or comparator) available in the stock.

346. **Drug Master File**
Refer to a compilation of data on the manufacturing, processing, packaging and storing of human drugs for regulatory submission.

347. **Drug Metabolism**
Refer to the pharmacokinetics of a drug substance.

348. **Drug Product**
A dosage form (*e.g.*, tablet, capsule, or suspension) that contains one or more drug substance.

349. **Drug Selection**
A drug discovery approach that involves finding a drug or group of drugs which works on the selected target.

350. **Due Diligence**
Refer to the verification of a person, document, process or activity.

351. **Dummy-*runs***
Refer to the mock runs for any activity or process before performing it in a real-time environment.

352. **Duration**
Refer to time scale.

6

E

353. Effective Dose
Refer to the dose of a drug substance that produces the desired efficacy outcome.

354. Efficacy
A product's ability to produce beneficial effects for a disease.

355. Electronic Data Capturing (EDC)
Use of electronic media (*e.g.* internet) for capturing trial data in pre-designed standard formats (case report forms).

356. Electronic Data Management (EDM)
Use of electronic media (*e.g.* internet) for capturing trial data in pre-designed standard formats followed by validation.

357. Electronic Form
Refer to pre-designed forms for recording trial data directly in to an electronic system.

358. Electronic Record
Any combination of text, graphics, data, audio, pictorial or other information representation in digital form that is created, modified, maintained, archived, retrieved or distributed by a computer system.

359. Electronic Signature
A computer data compilation of any symbol or series of symbols executed, adopted, or authorized by an individual to be the legal binding equivalent of the individual's handwritten signature.

360. Eligibility Criteria
Refer to the inclusion/exclusion criteria that make a subject eligible for a clinical trial.

361. Embryo
Early stages of a developing organism (from conception to the eighth week of pregnancy.

362. Emergency Use IND
A type of non-commercial Investigational New Drug Application whereby Regulatory Authority can authorize immediate dispensing of a non-approved drug in a life-threatening situation when no standard acceptable therapy is available and there is not enough time to obtain the ethics committee clearance. It may also be referred to as Compassionate Use IND.

363. Emergency Room
A place where emergency treatment of illness or injury is provided.

364. **Employee's Qualification Review**
A process to ascertain that management of clinical trial(s) and associated processes utilizes qualified individuals.

365. **End-of-Study Visit Report**
A site visit report that is prepared at the time of site closure visit(s).

366. **Endpoint**
An outcome or event to answer the primary hypothesis of a clinical trial.

367. **Enrolment Log**
Refer to a log that captures the dates of enrolment and other protocol required visits of a clinical trial subject.

368. **Entry Criteria**
Refer to the inclusion criteria that make a subject eligible for a clinical trial.

369. **Epidemiology**
The branch of medical science that deals with the study of incidence, distribution and control of a disease in a population.

370. **Equipoise**
Refer to a state of being balanced or in equilibrium.

371. **Equitable**
Refer to a state of being fair so that the benefits and burdens of research are fairly distributed.

372. **Equivalence and Non-inferiority**
Randomized trial design intended to establish that a new treatment has a similar rather than superior effect to an active control treatment. For equivalence studies, the intent is to establish that the difference between the new treatment and control is not large in either direction, whereas for non-inferiority studies the intent is to establish that the difference is not large in the direction favoring the control arm.

373. **Equivalence Studies**
Randomized trial design intended to establish that a new treatment has a similar rather than superior effect to an active control treatment. For equivalence studies, the intent is to establish that the difference between the new treatment and control is not large in either direction, *e.g.* bioequivalence studies.

374. **Essential Clinical Trial Documents**
Documents which individually and collectively permit evaluation of the conduct of a study and the quality of the data produced.

375. **Ethics**
Conforming to an accepted standard of human behavior.

376. **Ethics Advisory Board**
An independent body (a review board or a committee), constituted of medical

professionals and non-medical members, whose responsibility is to ensure the protection of the rights, safety and well being of human subjects involved in a clinical trial and to provide public assurance of that protection, by, among other things, reviewing and approving/providing favorable opinion on, the trial protocol, the suitability of the investigator(s), facilities, and the methods and material to be used in obtaining and documenting informed consent of the trial subjects. It may also be referred as Institutional Review Board (IRB), Institutional Ethics Committee (IEC) and Ethics Review Board (ERB).

377. **Ethics Review Board (ERB)**
Same as Ethics Advisory Board.

378. **European Union**
Organization of European countries dedicated to increasing economic integration and strengthening cooperation among its members.

379. **Evaluable**
Refer to a subject who has satisfied all the protocol requirements and is eligible for the safety and efficacy analysis.

380. **Exclusion Criteria**
Refer to the criteria that make a subject ineligible for a clinical trial.

381. **Exemptions**
Refer to the waivers that are provided under special circumstances with appropriate documentation of the authorization.

382. **Expected Event**
An event or outcome to answer the primary hypothesis of a clinical trial.

383. **Expedited Review**
Review for certain types of research involving no more than minimal risk and for minor changes in approved research which may be done solely by the chairperson of ethics committee or designee.

384. **Experimental Drug/ Investigational Product (IP)**
A pharmaceutical form of an active ingredient or placebo being tested or used as a reference in a clinical trial including a product with a marketing authorization when used or assembled (formulate or packaged) in a way different from the approved form or when used for an unapproved indication or when used to gain further information about an approved use.

385. **Experimental Study**
Any investigation in human subjects intended to discover or verify the clinical, pharmacological and/or other pharmacodynamic effects of an investigational product(s), and/or to identify any adverse reactions, and/or to study absorption, distribution, metabolism, and excretion of an investigational product(s) with the object of ascertaining its safety and efficacy.

386. **Explanatory Trial**
Refer to a clinical study designed to demonstrate the efficacy of a product.

387. **Extension Labeling**
Extension of expiry date on the label of an investigational product based on the available analysis/potency data.

388. **External Quality Review Organization**
Refer to an independent organization for reviewing the conduct of a clinical trial as per the pre-set quality standards.

389. **Extramural Research**
Refer to the research in an institution that is supported by external funding/grants instead of the in-house funding.

390. **E-submission**
Refer to submission to regulatory authorities via computer files.

7

F

391. **Fabrication**
Recording of false data or results and reporting them.

392. **Facility**
Refer to a place or site where clinical trials are conducted.

393. **Factorial Designs**
A special type of multi-arm trial that allows more than one comparison to be carried out without increasing the required sample size. The most common factorial design is 2x2 designs to compare two new treatments to no treatment (or placebo).

394. **False Negatives**
A result or finding which suggests that an observation (*e.g.* disease, response *etc.*) is not present but which, on further investigation is found to be present.

395. **False Positives**
A result or finding which suggests the presence of an observation (*e.g.* disease, response *etc.*) which turns out not to be there.

396. **Falsification**
Same as Fabrication.

397. **Familial/Social relations**
Relationships of significance in the life of a research subject such as parent-child, spousal, employer-employee.

398. **Family Member**
A legally competent person to take decision about a subject's medical care.

399. **Fatal Event**
An event resulting in death of a subject.

400. **FDA**
Food and Drug Administration that enforces laws governing food, drug, cosmetics and related public health laws.

401. **FDA 1572**
A list of commitments and requirements by the FDA for each investigator performing drug/biologics studies.

402. **FDA Oversight**
Supervision of clinical trials by Food and Drug Administration.

403. **Field Edit Description**
Refer to the validation applied for individual data field in the data management platform.

404. Federal Register
The official daily publication for rules, proposed rules, and notices of Federal agencies and organizations in United States.

405. Fetus
Later stages of a developing organism (from conception to delivery).

406. Final Report
Refer to the clinical study report prepared at the end (completion or termination) of a clinical trial.

407. Final Trial Close-Out Monitoring Report
A site visit report that is prepared after the site close-out visit.

408. Financial Disclosure
A form signed by Investigators and sub-investigators to disclose their financial interest in the Sponsor company for whom they intent to participate in the clinical trial.

409. Financial Planning
Refer to the panning of cost required to carry out a particular activity.

410. First-in-Human Study
Refer to Phase-1 clinical trial where the drug is first tested in human beings for its safety.

411. First-in-Man Study
Refer to Phase-1 clinical trial where the drug is first tested in human beings for its safety.

412. Fisher's Exact Test
A statistical test to determine whether there is a difference between two population groups in the proportion of subjects having a specified outcome. This is applicable only in a 2-by-2 table where there are 2 outcome categories and 2 population groups. For *e.g.* a study that compares the proportion of patients who had a particular pre-existing condition.

413. Follow-up Report
A report/response to provide additional information, clarification, or corrections to a previous report.

414. Food Drug and Cosmetic Act (FD and C Act)
A regulation applicable to the manufacture, sale, distribution, storage, import, export *etc.* of food, drug or cosmetic products.

415. Form G
A form about the rights of parents (of school children) regarding reviewing, amending and disclosing educational records.

416. Formulary
Refer to a list of drugs and their proper dosages to be used in a particular health plan.

417. Formulary Drugs
Same as Formulary.

418. **Formulation**
Refer to the mixture of chemicals and/or biological substances and excipients for preparing a dosage form.

419. **Fraud**
Misconduct such as falsification of data with a malicious intent.

420. **F-Test for ANOVA**
A statistical test to determine whether the mean value of a numeric variable (or response variable) is the same in each of different population groups. For *e.g.* a study that investigate whether the mean change in hemoglobin level after 12 weeks of treatment is different for patients treated with placebo and two different formulations of active drug.

421. **Full Board Review**
Refer to the ethics committee review that requires a full 'quorum' to be present for review.

G

422. Gene Therapy
Therapy that alters the genetic structure of cells for treating genetic diseases.

423. General Practitioner
A physician whose practice is not limited to a specialty.

424. Generic Drug
A medicinal product with the same active ingredient to an innovator drug.

425. Genetic Screening
Refer to the screening tests to identify if a person has an inherited predisposition to a certain phenotype or is at risk of producing offspring with inherited diseases or disorders.

426. Genotype
Refer to the genetic constitution of an individual.

427. Good Clinical Practice
Ethical and scientific quality standards for designing, conducting, recording and reporting trials that involves participation of human subjects.

428. Good Laboratory Practice
A standard for the conduct and reporting of non-clinical laboratory studies intended to assure the quality and integrity of safety data submitted to regulatory authorit.

429. Good Manufacturing Practice
A standard governing the manufacture of human and animal drugs and biologics intended to assure the quality and integrity of manufacturing data submitted to regulatory authorities.

430. Grants
Refer to the financial assistance provided by the funding agency/Sponsor to carry out a research project.

431. Grantee
Refer to the organization or individual who have been awarded a grant and is accountable for the use of the funds provided and for the performance of the a project or activities.

432. Graphical Presentation
Refer to the presentation of trial data in graphical forms (bar graphs, pie-charts *etc.*).

433. Group Sequential Design
Refer to a trial design that allows review of data at a particular time point based on formulating a stopping rule derived from repeated significance tests.

434. Guardian

An individual who is legally authorized to consent on behalf of a child for participation in a clinical trial.

435. Guidelines

Refer to a document that aims to streamline processes according to a set routine.

H

9

436. Half-life
Refer to the time required to eliminate 50% of the drug contained in the body.

437. Handling Instructions
Refer to the instructions needed to ensure proper storage, packaging, dispensing and disposition of investigational products.

438. Handwritten Signatures
The scripted name of an individual handwritten by that individual and executed or adopted with the intention to authenticate writing in a permanent form.

439. Harmonized Standard
Refer to the unified standards that are acceptable to all the participants.

440. Hazard Function
For an individual the probability of an event at a particular time given that the individual has survived to that time.

441. Health Authority
The regulatory authority in any country that frames policies and laws pertaining to drugs, biologics, devices and clinical trials.

442. Health Care
Refer to the services, care and supplies related to the health of an individual.

443. Health Care Agent
Legally authorized representative to make health decisions.

444. Health Care Clearinghouse
Public or private entities that either process or facilitate the processing of health information received from another entity into standard data elements or a standard transaction.

445. Health Care Provider
Any person, business, or agency that receives payment for health care in the normal course of business.

446. Health Insurance Portability and Accountability Act
Refer to United States legislation of 1996 (privacy rules effective April 14, 2003) that requires health care providers and others to obtain written authorization from patients or their legally authorized representatives before using or disclosing their Protected Health Information (PHI) for purposes other than treatment, billing, quality assurance and education.

447. **Health Level 7 (HL 7)**
A clinical data interchange messaging system in which messages are structured according to a pre-defined format and sent from one system to another.

448. **Health Maintenance Organization**
Refer to a medical group practice plan that acts both as an insurer and health care provider.

449. **Health Plan**
An individual or group plan that provides or pays the cost of medical care listed in government programs/rules.

450. **Healthy Volunteer**
Refer to an individual who participates in a Phase-1 clinical trial or a BA/BE study.

451. **Heterogeneity**
Refer to the variability or differences between the results of studies included in a systematic review.

452. **Heterologous**
Refer to organisms of a different but related species.

453. **Hierarchical Testing**
Testing that assigns an order of importance for the variables to be analyzed. Each analysis is performed according to this pre-specified hierarchy; however an analysis is only performed if the previous analysis was found to be statistically significant.

454. **High Performance Liquid Chromatography**
Refer to a form of liquid chromatography used to separate compounds that are dissolved in a solution.

455. **High Throughput Screening**
A drug discovery approach that involves testing the potential drug substances (obtained from massive compound libraries) against the target using automated robotic technology. High Throughput Screening yields hit compounds that are further studies for their physical, chemical and biological properties.

456. **HIPAA Authorization Form**
An authorization for the use and disclosure of protected health information.

457. **Histograms**
A display of the shape of distribution for numeric variables useful for examining a single numeric variable.

458. **Historical Control**
Refer to the use of available published data (historical data) as a control arm.

459. **Hit Compound**
Compounds obtained from High Throughput Screening process that demonstrates the ability to interact with the desired target.

460. Homebound
Refer to a condition of being confined to home and requiring considerable efforts and assistance to leave the home.

461. Homogeneity
Refer to the degree to which the results of studies included in a systematic review are similar.

462. Hospice
Refer to a program that provides special care for people who are near the end of life and for their families either at home, independent facilities or within hospitals.

463. Hospice Care
Refer to the palliative care for people who are near the end of life either at home, independent facilities or within hospitals.

464. Hospital
Refer to a health facility where sick or injured people are given medical or surgical care.

465. Human Subject
A patient or healthy individual who participates in a research study. Also referred to as study subjects.

466. Hybrid Entity
A single legal entity that uses or discloses protected health information only for a part of its business operations.

467. Hydration
Refer to the level of fluid in human body.

468. Hypothesis
Scientific rationale of a clinical trial.

10

I

469. ICH-GCP
International ethical and scientific quality standards for designing, conducting, recording and reporting trials that involves participation of human subjects.

470. Impartial Witness
Refer to a person who is independent of the trial and who witness the adequacy of informed consent process if the subject and/or his/her legally acceptable representative are unable to read and write.

471. Implant
A device that is placed permanently into a tissue or surgically formed cavity of the human body.

472. Incapacity
A state in which a person is no longer able to manage his or her affairs due to a physical or mental disability.

473. Incidence Rate
Refer to the number of new events in a population during a specified period of time.

474. Inclusion Criteria
Refer to the entry criteria that make a subject eligible for a clinical trial.

475. Incompetence
Same as Incapacity.

476. Investigational New Drug (IND)
Refer to a drug that is allowed to be used in clinical trials but not approved for marketing by a regulatory authority.

477. Indemnification
A legal statement or document indicating protection or exemption from liability for compensation or damages from a third party.

478. Indemnification Letter
A legal statement or document indicating protection or exemption from liability for compensation or damages from a third party.

479. Independent Data Monitoring Committee (IDMC)
Refer to an independent data-monitoring committee established by the sponsor to assess at intervals the progress of a clinical trial, the safety data, critical efficacy endpoints and to recommend to the sponsor whether to continue, modify or stop a trial.

480. Independent Ethics Committee
An independent body (a review board or a committee), constituted of medical

professionals and non-medical members, whose responsibility is to ensure the protection of the rights, safety and well being of human subjects involved in a clinical trial and to provide public assurance of that protection, by, among other things, reviewing and approving/providing favorable opinion on, the trial protocol, the suitability of the investigator(s), facilities, and the methods and material to be used in obtaining and documenting informed consent of the trial subjects.

481. Indication
Refer to a condition that forms the basis for the initiation of a treatment or of a diagnostic test.

482. Ineligibility
Refer to a condition in which a subject is not eligible for participation in a clinical trial.

483. Information Technology
Refer to the application of computer, communication and software technology for the management, processing and dissemination of information.

484. Informed Consent
A process by which a subject voluntarily confirms his or her willingness to participate in a particular trial after having been informed of all aspects of the trial that is relevant to subject's decision to participate. It is documented by means of a written, signed and dated informed consent form.

485. Informed Consent Document (ICD)
A document that describes the rights of the study participants and includes details about the study such as its purpose, duration, required procedures, risks, potential benefits and key contacts.

486. Informed Consent Form
Same as Informed Consent Document.

487. Infrastructure
Refer to the facility, equipments, personnel and processes required to carry out a clinical trial.

488. In-house Audit
Refer to a systematic examination of trial related activities and documents to determine whether the evaluated trial related activities were conducted, and the data were recorded, analyzed and accurately reported according to the protocol, sponsor's standard operating procedures (SOP), Good Clinical Practices (GCP) and the applicable regulatory requirements.

489. Innovative Therapy
Refer to a novel therapy backed by strong scientific data.

490. Inpatient Care
Refer to the care provided to patients when they are admitted to a hospital or health care centre.

491. **Inpatient Hospital Services**
Refer to the services (such nursing, dietary, diagnostic, medical and surgical services) offered to a patient who is admitted in a hospital.

492. **Inpatient Hospitalization**
Refer to a condition that requires admission to a hospital for its management.

493. **Inspection**
An official review of documents, facilities, records and any other resources related to a clinical trial by the regulatory authority at the site of the trial, at the sponsor's and/or contract research organization's (CRO's) facilities, or at other establishments deemed appropriate by the regulatory authority.

494. **Institution**
Any public or private entity or agency or medical or dental facility where clinical trials are conducted.

495. **Institutional Review Committee**
An independent body (a review board or a committee), constituted of medical professionals and non-medical members, whose responsibility is to ensure the protection of the rights, safety and well being of human subjects involved in a clinical trial and to provide public assurance of that protection, by, among other things, reviewing and approving/providing favorable opinion on, the trial protocol, the suitability of the investigator(s), facilities, and the methods and material to be used in obtaining and documenting informed consent of the trial subjects.

496. **Insurance Statement**
A legal statement that compensation for injuries related to trial drug or procedure will be available where required.

497. **Integrity**
An assurance about the authenticity, accuracy and validity of trial data.

498. **Intent-to-treat**
The intent-to-treat principle of statistical analysis in randomized trials states that all randomized patients should be included in the analysis and for the purposes of the analysis all patients should be included in the treatment group to which they were randomized even if they never received the treatment.

499. **Interaction**
The situation in which a treatment outcome (*e.g.* difference between investigational product and control) is dependent on another factor (*e.g.* Food-Drug interaction, Drug-Drug interaction *etc.*).

500. **Interactive Voice Response System (IVRS)**
An automated interactive voice response system used to randomize or withdraw the patients in a clinical trial.

501. **Interim Analysis**
Refer to the statistical analysis of trial data at a pre-defined time interval before all

subjects have completed the trial.

502. **Interim Clinical Trial/Study Report**
A report of intermediate results and their evaluation based on analyses performed during the course of a trial.

503. **Interim Data Lock**
Refer to the cleaning and locking of trial data for the purpose of interim analysis.

504. **Interim Report**
Refer to the report prepared after interim analysis of data.

505. **Internal Consistency**
Refer to the extent to which tests or procedures assess the same characteristic, skill or quality.

506. **Internet**
Refer to the global network of computers running internet protocol that provides the infrastructure for e-mail and other online activities.

507. **Inter-quartile Range**
The difference between upper and lower quartiles. It captures the variation in middle (50%) of data.

508. **Interval Data**
A continuous data where differences are interpretable but where there is no 'natural' zero. A good example is temperature in Fahrenheit degrees.

509. **Interval Scale**
A scale for ranking items where the distance between adjacent points are equal.

510. **Intervention**
Primary object of a clinical trial (*e.g.* Drug, Vaccine, Behavior, Device or Procedure).

511. **Invasive**
A medical procedure in which a part of the body is entered by puncture or incision.

512. **Invention**
Refer to discovery of a new drug, device, method, process or useful improvement upon any of these.

513. **Inventory**
Refer to the quantity of goods and materials available in the stock.

514. *In-vitro*
Refer to an artificial environment outside the living organism.

515. *In-vitro* **Fertilization**
Fertilization of an egg in an artificial environment (such as a laboratory dish or test tube) outside the living organism.

516. *In-vitro* **Testing**
Non-clinical testing conducted in an artificial environment (such as a test tube or

culture medium).

517. *In-vivo*
Refer to an environment inside the living organism.

518. *In-vivo* **Testing**
Testing conducted inside the living organism.

519. **Investigational Agent**
Refer to a pharmaceutical form of an active ingredient or placebo being tested or used as a reference in a clinical trial including a marketed product when used in an unapproved indication or dosage form.

520. **Investigational Device**
Refer to a device being tested in an investigation.

521. **Investigational Device Exemption (IDE)**
Refer to exemption (from Food, Drug and Cosmetics Act) to study investigational medical devices.

522. **Investigational Drug**
Same as Investigational Agent.

523. **Investigational New Drug Application (IND)**
Application filed by a drug sponsor to the FDA to obtain approval for human testing of its drug product.

524. **Investigational Plan**
A plan to define the objective, design, methodology, statistical considerations and organization of a trial.

525. **Investigational Product**
Refer to a pharmaceutical form of an active ingredient or placebo being tested or used as a reference in a clinical trial including a marketed product when used in an unapproved indication or dosage form.

526. **Investigational Site**
Refer to a medical facility where clinical trials are conducted.

527. **Investigator**
Refer to a person who is responsible for the conduct of a clinical trial at a site.

528. **Investigator Files**
Refer to the compilation of essential trial documents at a trial site.

529. **Investigator IND**
A type of non-commercial Investigational New Drug Application submitted by a physician who both initiates and conducts an investigation and under whose immediate direction the investigational drug is administered or dispensed.

530. **Investigator Master File**
Refer to a file that contains all the essential trial documents at a trial site.

531. **Investigator Meeting**
A meeting conducted before initiating a clinical trial for the uniform understanding of the protocol, processes and trial logistics among all the participating trial sites.

532. **Investigator Selection**
Refer to the process of selecting a suitable investigator for the conduct of a clinical trial.

533. **Investigator Site Approval**
A process of approving the selection of a suitable investigator for the conduct of a clinical trial.

534. **Investigator Site Assessment Report**
A detailed report (prepared after reviewing the Investigator's qualification, site's infrastructure, documentation practices, storage and archival system *etc.*) which forms the basis for the selection of potential Investigator(s).

535. **Investigator Site Evaluation**
Refer to the process of evaluating a suitable investigator for the conduct of a clinical trial.

536. **Investigator Site File**
Refer to a file that contains all the essential trial documents at a trial site.

537. **Investigator Training**
Refer to imparting training on study protocol, trial procedures and processes to the investigator.

538. **Investigator Undertaking**
A formal written, commitment (submitted to regulatory authorities) by trial investigator(s) assuring their compliance with the study protocol and all the applicable regulatory requirements.

539. **Investigator's Brochure**
A compilation of the clinical and non-clinical data on the investigational product(s).

540. **Investigator's Qualification**
Qualification of a clinical trial investigator documented in the form of a curriculum vitae.

541. **Investigational Product (IP) Accountability Logs**
A document/log to record receipt, dispensing, return and destruction of IP in order to ascertain 100% accountability.

542. **IP Destruction Certificate**
A document that lists the quantities of IP (both used and unused) destroyed at the end of the trial or at a specified interval.

J

543. Job Description

A document that lists the core job functions of a job.

544. Justice

Refer to the principle of moral rightness in action or attitude.

K

545. Kaplan-Meier Estimate

An estimate for the survivor function.

546. Kruskal-Wallis Test

A statistical test that provides an analysis of variance by ranks and is the non-parametric equivalent of the F-test for analysis of variance. This test requires the presence of 3 or more comparison groups. For *e.g.* A study that investigate the number of hypoglycemic episodes per patient between three groups of patients on different insulin formulations.

L

547. Label
Refer to a document for identifying a drug/placebo in compliance with applicable regulations and appropriateness of the instructions provided to the subjects.

548. Labeling
Refer to the process of applying label to a drug/placebo.

549. Laboratory
Refer to a facility which performs testing (*e.g.* biochemical, microbiological, serological, chemical, immunohematological, biophysical, cytological, pathological *etc.*) on specimens derived from humans for providing information on the diagnosis, prevention, treatment of disease or assessment of overall health.

550. Laboratory Accreditation
Refer to the act of granting recognition to a laboratory for maintaining suitable standards and processes.

551. Laboratory Alerts
Refer to the act of highlighting out of range laboratory values.

552. Laboratory Certification
Same as Laboratory Accreditation.

553. Laboratory Data
Refer to results or reports of laboratory tests.

554. Laboratory Kits
Refer to pre-labeled kits containing empty containers/vacutainers for collection of desired biological specimen (*e.g.* blood, serum, plasma, urine, saliva *etc.*).

555. Laboratory Normal Ranges
Refer to the normal value ranges for standardized laboratory tests.

556. Laboratory Reference Ranges
Refer to the normal value ranges for standardized laboratory tests.

557. Laboratory Report
Refer to a document that contains results of the laboratory tests for a specific subject.

558. Lactation
Refer to the period of time during which a woman is providing her breast milk to an infant or child.

559. Lead Candidates
Hit compounds (compounds that demonstrates the ability to interact with the desired

target) with suitable physical, chemical and biological properties.

560. **Lead Molecule**
Same as Lead Candidates.

561. **Lead Optimization**
The process of modifying the lead candidates by combinatorial chemistry to produce a large number of variants for further pre-clinical and clinical testing.

562. **Legally Acceptable Representative (LAR)**
An individual or juridical or other body authorized under applicable law to consent for the subject's participation in the clinical trial on behalf of a prospective subject.

563. **Legally Authorized Representative (LAR)**
Same as Legally Acceptable Representative.

564. **Letter of Confidentiality (LOC)**
A document that establishes agreement between two or more parties for ensuring the confidentiality of information provided by one party to the other. It may also be called as Confidentiality Agreement or Non Disclosure Agreement (NDA).

565. **License**
An official or legal permission to an individual or organization by a competent authority to engage in a practice, occupation or activity.

566. **Life-threatening Adverse Drug Experience**
Refer to an adverse drug experience in which a subject is at immediate risk of dying.

567. **Line Extension**
Refer to investigation of an approved drug in a new/unapproved indication.

568. **Line Management**
Refer to organizational hierarchical structure of the supervisors and the subordinates.

569. **Listed Drug**
Refer to drugs that have marketing authorization and can be sold in a country.

570. **Letter of Agreement (LOA)**
Refer to a legal agreement between two or more parties that specifies the scope of work, obligations and payment schedule.

571. **Local Area Network (LAN)**
Refer to a local computer network for communication between computers in a limited physical area.

572. **Logistics Planning and Management**
Refer to the planning, organization and management of trial logistics such as shipment of investigational product and other supplies, central lab/radiology services, refrigerated shipment of biological specimens *etc.*

573. **Lost to Follow-up**
Refer to a trial subject who is not traceable by any means before completion of his/her participation in the trial.

14

M

574. **Management of Adverse Events**
Medical management of an adverse event and its reporting to the applicable regulatory authorities within the stipulated time-frame.

575. **Manuscript**
Refer to articles that are published in peer-reviewed scientific Journals.

576. **Marketing Application**
Refer to the application filed for seeking marketing authorization of a new drug/device.

577. **Master Randomization List**
Refer to the master list that captures the distribution schedule of trial subjects between treatment and control arm.

578. **Master Subject Log**
Refer to the master list/log that captures the names and other identifiers of trial subjects.

579. **Matched Pair**
A type of parallel trial design in which investigator(s) identify pairs of subjects who are identical with respect to relevant factors, then randomize them so that one receives a treatment and the other receives another treatment.

580. **Matrices Tracking**
Refer to the review of planned matrices (such as subject enrolment, trial milestones *etc.*) versus actual figures.

581. **Maximum Tolerated Dose**
The highest daily dose of a chemical that does not causes overt toxicity in a ninety-day study in laboratory mice or rats.

582. **McNemar's Test**
A statistical test to determine whether there is an association between two categorical variables when the data are paired. For *e.g.* a cross-over study where patients are required to provide their assessment about the response during each treatment period.

583. **Mean**
An arithmetic value that is obtained by summing up all the observations and dividing the total by the total number of observations.

584. **Measurement**
A process of estimating the magnitude of some attributes of an object such as its length or weight.

585. **Mechanism of Action**
The explanation of the mechanism by which a drug produces an effect in a living

organism.

586. **Me Watch Form**
Refer to the safety narratives prepared from a serious adverse event.

587. **Median**
The middle most observation. It is a better indication of central value when one or more of the lowest or highest observations are wide apart.

588. **Median Survival Time**
The time at which 50% of the study population is alive.

589. **Medical Advisor**
Medically qualified personnel in an organization who supports marketing and/or research department.

590. **Medical Device**
An instrument, apparatus, machine, implant or other similar or related article including any component, part or accessory which is intended for use in the diagnosis, cure, treatment or prevention of disease.

591. **Medical Dictionary for Regulatory Activities (MedDRA)**
A standardized dictionary of medical terminology adopted by the International Conference on Harmonization.

592. **Medical Doctor**
A person who is eligible to undertake medical practice as per the applicable regulations.

593. **Medical History**
The information on overall general health, past illnesses and current medical problems of a subject.

594. **Medical License**
An authorization to undertake medical practice as per applicable regulations.

595. **Medical Monitor**
A medically qualified personnel employed by trial Sponsors/CROs for reviewing critical medical data (safety and efficacy) of a clinical trial.

596. **Medical Records**
Original documents, data, and records (*e.g.* hospital records, clinical and office charts, laboratory notes, memoranda, subject's diaries or evaluation checklists, pharmacy dispensing records, recorded data from automated instruments, copies or transcriptions certified after verification as being accurate and complete, microfiches, photographic negatives, microfilms or magnetic media, X-rays, subject's files, and records kept at the pharmacy, at the laboratories, and at medico-technical departments involved in the clinical trial).

597. **Medication**
Refer to articles (other than food) intended for the use in the diagnosis, cure, mitigation,

treatment or prevention of disease in man or other animals.

598. **Mega Trials**
Large scale clinical trials having a sample size of 10,000 or more that evaluates the marginally effective investigational product.

599. **Memorandum of Understanding**
A formal written agreement which sets forth the working arrangements between two or more groups.

600. **Mentally Disabled**
A state in which a person is not able to manage his or her affairs or to make a choice due to a psychiatric or developmental disorder.

601. **Meta-Analysis**
Meta-analysis combines the results of several studies that address a set of related research hypotheses. It is widely used in epidemiology and evidence-based medicine studies.

602. **Metabolism**
A process by which a drug substance is changed by the body and converted in to more polar, hydrophilic compounds which the body can excrete more easily.

603 **Microfiche**
An archival media on which essential trial documents can be transferred at a very small size (miniaturize form).

604. **Milestones**
Refer to an objective or goal to be achieved in a stipulated timeframe.

605. **Minimal Risk**
The extent of harm or discomfort anticipated from a clinical trial/research which is not greater than the routine practice.

606. **Minimum Effective Dose**
Minimal concentration level at which a drug is able to produce an effect in human body.

607. **Minor**
An individual who has not attained the legal age of consenting to a trial as per the applicable regulations.

608. **Minutes of Meeting**
A document that summarize the critical discussion and decision points of a meeting.

609. **Misconduct**
Refer to the fabrication or falsification of data in reporting results of a clinical trial.

610. **Mode**
A most frequently occurring value in a set of data.

611. **Modem**
Refer to a device that converts digital data into analog data.

612. Modification

The act of making change or amendment to an information, document or process.

613. Molecular Modeling

A technique to generate 3D structures of target molecules and model the affinity of different molecules at these targets using powerful software graphics and simulation programs.

614. Monitor

A person employed by the Sponsor or CRO who reviews study records to determine that a study is being conducted in accordance with the protocol and applicable regulatory guidelines.

615. Monitoring

The act of overseeing the progress of a clinical trial and of ensuring that it is conducted, recorded and reported in accordance with the protocol, Standard Operating Procedures (SOPs), Good Clinical Practice (GCP) and the applicable regulatory requirement(s).

616. Monitoring Visit Report

A written report prepared by the monitor after each site visit to document the progress and conduct of the trial at a site.

617. Monitoring Plan

A document that specifies the monitoring visit interval, source data verification requirements and protocol specific monitoring instructions.

618. Monitoring Report

Same as Monitoring Visit Report.

619. Monitoring Visit

Same as Monitoring.

620. Monitoring Visit Log

A log signed by the monitor each time he/she visits the trial site.

621. Morbidity

The frequency of a disease, illness, injury, and disability in a population.

622. Morbidity Rate

The rate of illness in a population.

623. Mortality Rate

The total number of deaths relative to the total population at a specific place in a specific period of time.

624. Multi-arm Parallel Designs

A type of parallel design that compares more than two treatments. It has an advantage of simultaneously being able to compare more than one treatment to a placebo arm, and also to compare two alternative new therapies.

625. **Multi-centre Trial**
A clinical trial conducted according to a single protocol but at more than one site by more than one investigator.

626. **Multi-centric Trial**
Same as Multi-centre Trial.

627. **Mutagenic Studies**
A type of *in vivo* and *in vitro* toxicological testing of 18-24 months duration to determine the mutagenic potential of a drug.

628. NCR Paper
Refer to No Carbon Required paper (a special paper mostly used in CRFs that does not require a carbon sheet for getting a carbon copy).

629. Non Disclosure Agreement (NDA)
A document that establishes agreement between two or more parties for ensuring the confidentiality of information provided by one party to the other.

630. Neglect
Refer to willful oversight in performing a particular activity.

631. Neonate
Refer to newborn baby.

632. New Chemical Entity
Refer to chemical molecule that after undergoing clinical trials could translate into a potential drug for the cure/treatment of a disease.

633. New Drug Application
An application submitted by the manufacturer of a drug to the FDA after Phase 3 trials for obtaining marketing authorization of a new drug.

634. New Molecular Entity
Same as New Chemical Entity.

635. N-of-1 Design
A type of clinical trial design that is carried out in a single patient. Such designs are related to cross-over designs and involve treatment comparisons within the same individual based on an outcome observed repeatedly over time. It is appropriate for chronic conditions involving treatments that lead to immediate transient effects such as pain relief.

636. No Action Indicated
A classification of regulatory inspection outcome that does not require any action or response.

637. No Treatment Control
Refer to subject who are randomly assigned to the no treatment arm in a clinical trial.

638. Nominal Data
Type of qualitative test or categorical data. For *e.g.* Sex: Male/Female; Treatment Group: A/B.

639. Non Clinical Study
Biomedical studies not performed on human subjects.

640. **Non Commercial IND**
A type of Investigational New Drug Application filed for carrying out non-commercial research. It includes Investigator IND, Emergency Use IND and Treatment IND.

641. **Non Comparative Study**
Refer to a trial design that does not have a comparative arm.

642. **Non Compliance**
Refer to the deviation from the protocol, standard operating procedures or applicable regulatory guidelines.

643. **Non Evaluable**
Refer to the subject(s) whose data can not be included in the safety and/or efficacy analysis.

644. **Non Governmental Organization (NGO)**
Refer to the non for profit charitable organization.

645. **Non-inferiority Studies**
Randomized trial design intended to establish that a new treatment has a similar rather than superior effect to an active control treatment. For non-inferiority studies the intent is to establish that the difference between the new treatment and control is not large in direction favoring the control arm *e.g.* bioequivalence studies.

646. **Non Invasive**
Refer to a medical procedure that does not involve skin break.

647. **Non Parametric Tests**
A distribution free test that is applied when the data is not normally distributed. It is used to compare observations repeated on the same subjects. For *e.g.* Mann-Whitney U test, Wilcoxon test, Krushall-Wallis test *etc.*

648. **Non Responder**
Refer to the subject(s) that does not respond to the trial drug or therapy.

649. **Non-significant**
Yielding a value from a statistical test that lies within the limits for being of random occurrence.

650. **Normal Lab Values**
Refer to the normal value ranges for standardized laboratory tests of any laboratory.

651. **Not Approvable Letter**
Refer to an action letter (after the review of a new drug application) which lists the deficiencies in the application and explains why the application can not be approved.

652. **Notes to File**
Refer to the notes to explain the deviation/violation of a particular activity/process.

653. **Notice of Inspection**
Refer to an official communication from regulatory agency to the investigator/sponsor

for undertaking a regulatory inspection.

654. Null Hypothesis

It is a statement claiming that a population parameter takes a specified value in accordance with an underlying theory about one or more populations. The null hypothesis posits equality (no difference) between the treatments and is denoted as H_0 as a standard statistical practice.

655. Numeric Data

Quantitative data such as number of patients, number of visits *etc.*

656. Numeric Continuous Data

A type of quantitative data. For *e.g.* Blood Pressure, Pulse Rate.

657. Numeric Discrete Data

A type of quantitative data. For *e.g.* Number of Children in a Family.

658. Nuremberg Code

As a result of the medical experimentation conducted by Nazis during World War II, the U.S. Military Tribunal in Nuremberg in 1947 set forth a code of medical ethics for researchers conducting clinical trials. The code is designed to protect the safety and integrity of study participants.

16

O

659. **Objective Measurement**
A measurement that yields a quantitative assessment.

660. **Observational Study**
A non-interventional study conducted according to routine medical practice.

661. **Odds Ratio (OR)**
Refer to the odds in favor of disease among exposed individuals divided by the odds in favor of disease among the unexposed individuals. It is the only parameter that can be used to compare two groups of binary data responses from a retrospective study.

662. **Off Label**
The unauthorized use of a drug for an indication which is not approved by the Regulatory Authorities.

663. **Office for Human Research Protection (OHRP)**
A federal government agency (in U.S.) that issues assurances and overseas compliance of regulatory guidelines by research institutions.

664. **Off Shoring**
Refer to the relocation of business processes from one country to another.

665. **Open Design**
Refer to a trial design in which all the involved parties (investigator, subject and monitor) know the treatment group to which a subject is assigned.

666. **Open Label**
Same as Open Design.

667. **Open System**
Refer to an environment in which system access is not controlled by persons who are responsible for the content of electronic records that are on the system.

668. **Operational Data Model (ODM)**
As defined by CDISC, "a vendor neutral, platform independent format for interchange and archive of data collected from various sources in clinical trials".

669. **Operating Manuals**
A reference document that contains operating instructions for an equipment, activity or process.

670. **Opinion Leader**
Refer to a subject matter expert in a peer-group.

671. **Oral Consent**
Refer to a verbal consent by a subject who is not in a position to provide written consent.

672. Ordinal Data

Type of qualitative or categorical data. For *e.g.* Severity of Disease: Mild/Moderate/Severe.

673. Organogram

Refer to an organizational chart that describes different functional positions in an organization.

674. Original Medical Record

Refer to original documents, data, and records (*e.g.* hospital records, clinical and office charts, laboratory notes, memoranda, subjects' diaries or evaluation checklists, pharmacy dispensing records, recorded data from automated instruments, copies or transcriptions certified after verification as being accurate copies, microfiches, photographic negatives, microfilm or magnetic media, X-rays, subject files, and records kept at the pharmacy, at the laboratories and at medico-technical departments involved in the clinical trial).

675. Orphan Drug

Refer to a designation of the FDA (in U.S.) to indicate a therapy developed to treat a rare disease (one which affects a U.S. population of less than 200,000 people).

676. Outcome

Refer to the result of an activity, process, investigation or intervention.

677. Outcome Data

Same as Outcome.

678. Outcome Indicator

Refer to an indicator for the assessment of outcome data.

679. Outcome Research

Refer to the measurement of the value of a particular course of therapy.

680. Outlier

Refer to an observation that is numerically distant (inconsistent) from rest of the data.

681. Outlier Detection

Data points which lay a long way from the main body of similar data.

682. Outpatient

Refer to the ambulatory care at a hospital that dose not require hospitalization.

683. Outsourcing

Refer to the transfer of a business activity/process to an external service provider.

684. Overhead

Refer to the operational expenses (*e.g.* electricity, rental *etc.*)

685. Over-the-Counter (OTC)

Drugs available for purchase without a physician's prescription.

17

P

686. Package Insert
Refer to a product information sheet that summarizes all the clinical and non-clinical information of a drug product.

687. Paired t-Tet
A statistical test to determine whether the mean change from baseline to endpoint of a numeric variable is different from zero. This test requires 1 population group with 2 measurements of the numeric variable per patient. For *e.g.* a study that investigates mean change in weight within a group of patients from baseline to endpoint.

688. Paper Flow
Refer to the step-by-step process to be followed from the data transcription in the Case Report Forms (CRFs) at the site to its collection, entry, validation and final analysis.

689. Paper Flow Process
Same as Paper Flow.

690. Paper Trail
Refer to the documentation of activities that allows reconstruction of the course of events.

691. Parallel Designs
A type of statistical design in which patients are randomized to one of two treatment strategies and the two arms are then prospectively followed in parallel throughout the trial.

692. Parallel Track
Refer to a system of making experimental drugs available to individuals who are unable to participate in clinical trials.

693. Parameter
Refer to a factor that defines a system and its performance.

694. Parametric Tests
A statistical test in which a sample statistics is obtained to estimate the population parameter. It is applied when the data is normally distributed. For *e.g.* ANOVA, t-Test *etc.*

695. Parent
Refer to a child's biological or adoptive parent.

696. Participant
Refer to a subject who takes part in a clinical trial.

697. **Patent**
Refer to a document that grants the sole right of an invention to its inventor.

698. **Patent Application**
Refer to an application filed to the concerned authorities for seeking patent for an invention.

699. **Patient**
Refer to an individual who required medical care or treatment.

700. **Patient Block**
Refer to a set of patient numbers that are grouped together for statistical purposes.

701. **Patient Cards**
Refer to a document given to the study subjects for recording certain observations/readings on the condition of their health either at home or at the trial site.

702. **Patient Diaries**
Same as Patient Cards.

703. **Patient File**
Refer to the hospital/clinic file that contains complete medical information of a patient/subject.

704. **Patient Number**
Refer to a unique numerical identifier assigned to a trial subject.

705. **Patient Recruitment**
Refer to the act of enrolling subject in a clinical trial.

706. **Patient Summary**
Refer to a document that summarizes the past and present medical health condition of a subject.

707. **Peer Review**
Review of a clinical trial data by experts chosen by the study sponsor. These experts review the trials for scientific merit, participant safety and ethical considerations.

708. **Percentiles**
Refer to values in a series of observations arranged in ascending order of magnitude which divide the distribution into 100 equal parts. Thus the median is 50th percentile. The 50th percentile will have 50% observations on either side. 10th percentile will have 10% observations to the left and 90% observations to the right.

709. **Performance Review**
Refer to the review of the performance of an individual in a specified period of time against pre-set objectives.

710. **Periodic Safety Update Report (PSUR)**
Refer to the safety reporting of marketed drugs in a specified period of time (generally on an annual basis).

711. **Permission**
Refer to the authorization granted by the regulatory authorities.

712. **Pharmaceutical Alternatives**
Refer to the drug products that contains the same therapeutic moiety but are different salts, dosage forms or strengths.

713. **Pharmaceutical Equivalents**
Refer to the drug products that have the same active ingredient, dosage form, route of administration, strength or concentration.

714. **Pharmacist**
Refer to a person qualified to prepare and dispense drugs and certified by concerned authority to do so.

715. **Pharmacodynamics**
Refer to the physiological effect of drug on human body.

716. **Pharmacoeconomics**
Refer to the study of cost-benefit ratio of drugs with other therapies or with similar drugs.

717. **Pharmacogenetics**
Refer to the study of genetic variation leading to differential response to drugs.

718. **Pharmacogenomics**
Refer to the study of genetic variation underlying differential response to drugs.

719. **Pharmacokinetics**
Refer to the process (in a living organism) of absorption, distribution, metabolism and excretion of a drug or vaccine.

720. **Pharmacological Testing**
Studies to explore the pharmacological activity and therapeutic potential of compounds. It involves the use of animals, isolated cell cultures and tissues, enzymes and cloned receptor sites as well as computer models.

721. **Pharmacology**
The study of the effect of drugs on living organism.

722. **Pharmacopoeia**
Refer to a reference book that contains official listing of marketed drugs.

723. **Pharmacovigilance**
Refer to the methods of assessment and prevention of adverse events.

724. **Pharmacy**
Refer to a place where drugs are prepared and dispensed.

725. **Phases of Clinical Trials**
Refer to different phases of drug development process after the pre-clinical

development of a drug candidate is completed. There are four phases of clinical trials Phase 1, 2, 3 and 4.

726. **Phase 0 Trial**

Refer to human microdosing studies designed to speed up the development of promising molecular entities or imaging agents by establishing (very early on) whether the drug or agent behaves in human subjects as was expected from preclinical studies through pharmacodynamic biomarker assays.

727. **Phase 1 Trial**

First in man studies to establish the initial safety, maximum tolerance, pharmacokinetics *etc.* in healthy human volunteers. For anti-cancer drugs Phase 1 studies are also carried out in patients.

728. **Phase 2 Trial**

Universally accepted as a standard requirement for the evaluation of efficacy and safety of the drug. Careful observations are made to determine the dose and adverse reactions in patients with the relevant indication.

729. **Phase 2a Trial**

Pilot clinical trials to evaluate safety in selected patient population.

730. **Phase 2b Trial**

Controlled clinical trials to evaluate safety and efficacy for determining a dose range to be studied in Phase-3 trials.

731. **Phase 3 Trial**

Final pre-marketing trial for evaluating the safety and efficacy of a drug in a large patient population. Phase 3 trial forms the basis of Regulatory submissions.

732. **Phase 3a Trial**

Conducted after the drug's efficacy is demonstrated but before the regulatory submission of New Drug Application (*e.g.* studies in children or patients with renal dysfunction *etc.*).

733. **Phase 3b Trial**

Conducted after regulatory submission but prior to the drug's approval or launch (*e.g.* to supplement or complement earlier trials).

734. **Phase 4 Trial**

Post marketing studies to collect the additional safety data from a much larger patient population.

735. **Phenotype**

Refer to any observable characteristic or trait of an organism such as morphology, biochemical or physiological properties.

736. **Physician**

Refer to a person authorized by law to practice medicine.

737. **Pie Charts**
Refer to a type of statistical chart that displays the distribution of levels of a categorical variable. It can display percentages or count.

738. **Pilot Study**
Refer to an initial study to explore new hypotheses.

739. **Pivotal Study**
Refer to a well controlled, randomized study to evaluate the safety and efficacy of a new drug in patients with relevant disease condition.

740. **Pivotal Trial**
Same as Pivotal Study.

741. **Placebo**
Refer to an inactive substance designed to resemble the drug being tested. It is used as a control to rule out any psychological effects.

742. **Placebo Controlled Study**
A method of investigation of drugs in which an inactive substance (the placebo) is given to one group of participants while the other group receives the investigational product. The results obtained in the two groups are then compared to see if the investigational treatment is more effective in treating the condition.

743. **Placebo Controlled Trial**
Same as Placebo Controlled Study.

744. **Placebo Effect**
Refer to the psychological effects of receiving a drug when no drug (or inactive substance) is administered to a patient.

745. **Plagiarism**
Refer to the act of copying someone's words, idea, results and presenting them as original content.

746. **Policies and Procedures**
Refer to the detailed, written instructions to achieve uniformity and consistency in the performance of a specific function.

747. **Policy**
Refer to the written instructions or rules to achieve uniformity, consistency and decision making.

748. **Portable Document Format (PDF)**
Refer to a file format created by Adobe Systems independent of the application software, hardware and operating system.

749. **Post Marketing Surveillance**
A systematic approach to collect the additional safety data on a drug from a much larger patient population once it is marketed.

750. Poster
Refer to a document to present the scientific results on a single sheet using text, figures, tables and graphs.

751. Potency
Refer to the concentration/strength of a drug at which it is effective.

752. Power and Sample Size
Refer to the likelihood that the study will reject the null hypothesis of no treatment difference when the truth is that the two treatments do differ. The power of a study is directly related to the number of patients in the study or the sample size. As the sample size increases the power also increases.

753. Power of Attorney
Refer to a legal document that allows a person to act on behalf of another person.

754. Practice
Refer to a fashion in which an activity is routinely performed.

755. Pragmatic Trial
Refer to a clinical trial designed to examine the benefits of a product under real-world environment.

756. Pre Clinical Study
Studies conducted either *in vitro* but usually *in vivo* on animals to determine that the drug is safe.

757. Pre Clinical Investigations
Investigation of the pharmacological activity of a new compound using a wide array of chemical and biochemical assays, cell-culture models and animal models in a laboratory.

758. Pre Clinical Testing
Same as Pre Clinical Investigations.

759. Pre-existing Conditions
Refer to the clinical complaints that a patient have at the time of entry into the study.

760. Pregnancy
Refer to the period from conception to birth.

761. Pre-mature Termination
Refer to terminating/stopping an activity before the planned completion time-frame.

762. Prescription
Written instructions by a doctor that contains the names of drugs along with the description of dosage form as well as directions for use.

763. Prescription Drug
Drugs that can be sold only through prescriptions.

764. **Pre-study Visit**
The initial visit to investigator site by the sponsor/CRO personnel in order to evaluate the suitability of investigator and facility for a trial.

765. **Pre-study Visit Report**
Refer to the written report that summarizes the observations and findings of pre-study visit.

766. **Pre-trial Monitoring Report**
Refer to the written report that summarizes the observations and findings of pre-study visit.

767. **Pre-trial Monitoring Visit**
The initial visit to investigator site by the sponsor/CRO personnel in order to evaluate the suitability of investigator and facility for a trial.

768. **Prevalence**
Refer to the number of people in a given population with a specific condition.

769. **Prevention Trial**
Refer to clinical trials that address new methods of preventing disease.

770. **Preventive Services**
Refer to health care services for the prevention of diseases.

771. **Primary Care Physician**
Refer to a doctor trained to provide basic medical care.

772. **Primary Outcome**
The actual occurrence of a primary event (*e.g.* cure, death *etc.*) in a clinical study patient.

773. **Principal Investigator**
Refer to a person responsible for the conduct of clinical trial at a trial site.

774. **Prisoner**
Refer to a person who is confined to custody.

775. **Privacy**
Refer to the state of being private.

776. **Private Information**
The personal information of an individual which is not known to others.

777. **Procedure**
A particular method of performing a task.

778. **Process**
A series of actions or events for performing a task.

779. **Process Deviation**
Refer to non-compliance to a process.

780. **Process Improvement**
The methods or steps that can improve an existing process in an efficient manner.

781. **Product Monograph**
A document that summarizes all the clinical and non-clinical information of a drug product.

782. **Project Management**
Methods used for planning, organizing and managing a clinical trial project.

783. **Project Plan**
A written plan to define the critical project milestones, cost estimate, timelines and deliverables.

784. **Prophylactic**
Refer to a preventive measure.

785. **Proposal**
Refer to a written description of a work plan.

786. **Proprietary**
Refer to ownership of sole rights of a document, process or product.

787. **Prospective Study**
A study that moves forward in time.

788. **Protected Health Information (PHI)**
Refer to any information about health status, provision of health care or payment for health care that can be linked to an individual.

789. **Protection of Pupil Rights Amendment (PPRA)**
Department of education regulation (in U.S.) that states that surveys, questionnaires and instructional materials for school children must be inspected by parents/guardians.

790. **Protocol**
A document that describes the objective(s), design, methodology, statistical considerations and organization of a trial. The protocol also gives the background rationale for the trial.

791. **Protocol Addendum**
Refer to the written supplement or additions to the approved protocol.

792. **Protocol Amendment**
Refer to the written description of a change(s) to or formal clarification of a protocol.

793. **Protocol Deviation**
Refer to non-compliance with the protocol schedule of events.

794. **Protocol Modification**
Refer to the written description of a change(s) to a protocol.

795. **Protocol Review Committee**
A core group within an institution or organization that reviews trial protocols for

completeness, accuracy, compliance and feasibility.

796. Protocol Signature Page
A document that acknowledges the investigator and/or sponsor agreement to the protocol.

797. Protocol Signature Sheet
Same as Protocol Signature Page.

798. Protocol Violation
Same as Protocol Deviation.

799. Proxy
Refer to a person authorized to act on behalf of another person.

800. Professional Services Agreement (PSA)
A written, dated and signed agreement between two or more parties that sets out any arrangements on delegation and distribution of tasks, obligations and if applicable on financial matters.

801. Publication
Refer to publishing the results of a clinical trial in a peer-reviewed Journal.

802. Purchase Order
A written authorization issued by a buyer to a seller, indicating the type, quantities and agreed prices for products or services.

803. Purity
Refer to the absence of extraneous material in a drug product.

804. p-Value
The probability that the observed discrepancy is simply a chance occurrence if in fact the null hypothesis is true. It is a standard practice to use the probability levels of 0.05 to represent the cut-off point that defines a high or low probability of a chance occurrence.

18

Q

805. **Qualitative Variable**
A variable that is based on categorical data and can not be measured numerically (*e.g.* gender, race).

806. **Quality**
Refer to a pre-set standard for measuring the outcome.

807. **Quality Assurance (QA)**
All those planned and systematic actions that are established to ensure that the trial is performed and the data are generated, documented (recorded) and reported in compliance with Good Clinical Practice (GCP) and the applicable regulatory requirement(s).

808. **Quality Assurance Report**
Refer to a written document that captures the observations and findings of quality assurance audit.

809. **Quality Assurance Unit**
Refer to an independent group of personnel to ensure that the trial is performed and the data are generated, documented (recorded) and reported in compliance with Good Clinical Practice (GCP) and the applicable regulatory requirement(s).

810. **Quality Control (QC)**
The operational techniques and activities undertaken within the quality assurance system to verify that the requirements for quality of the trial-related activities have been fulfilled.

811. **Quality Improvement**
Refer to the activities undertaken within the quality assurance system to identify the problems and examine the implementation of solutions.

812. **Quality Improvement Organization**
Refer to an organization that monitors the appropriateness, effectiveness and quality of care provided to Medicare beneficiaries.

813. **Quality of Life (QOL)**
Refer to an individual's sense of general well-being and ability to perform various tasks.

814. **Quality of Life Questionnaire(QLQ)**
Refer to a validated data collection form that contains a series of questions to assess an individual's sense of general well-being and ability to perform various tasks.

815. **Quality of Life Trials**
Refer to trials that explore ways to improve comfort and quality of life for individuals

with a chronic illness.

816. **Quality Review of Database**
The process of comparing case report form and ancillary data to the raw data in the clinical trial reporting database.

817. **Quantitative Variable**
A variable that is based on numerical data or can be measure numerically (*e.g.* weight, height, blood pressure).

818. **Quartiles**
These are three different points located on the entire range of a variable Q_1, Q_2 and Q_3. Q_1 or lower quartile will have 25% observations falling on its left and 75% on its right. Q_2 or median will have 50% observations on either side. Q_3 or upper quartile will have 75% observations on its left and 25% on its right.

819. **Quasi Experimental Study**
Refer to a study in which subjects are randomly assigned to groups by the experimenter according to a strict logic allowing causal inference about the effects of the interventions under investigation.

820. **Questionnaire**
Refer to a validated data collection form that contains a series of questions to assess an individual's response on a topic/parameter.

R

19

821. **Random**
Refer to an element of chance or having no specific pattern.

822. **Random Allocation**
Refer to the process of assigning trial subjects to treatment or control groups using an element of chance in order to reduce bias.

823. **Random Assignment**
Same as Random Allocation.

824. **Random Number Table**
Refer to a table obtained through statistical tests that contains randomization schedule.

825. **Random Sample**
Refer to a method of selection designed to ensure that each object has an equal chance of getting selected.

826. **Randomization**
Same as Random Allocation.

827. **Randomization Code**
Refer to a list that contains the randomization schedule of assigning trial subjects to treatment or control groups.

828. **Randomization List**
Same as Randomization Code.

829. **Randomized Control Trial**
Refer to a trial that randomly assign participants to an intervention group or to a control group in order to measure the effects of the intervention.

830. **Randomized Trial**
Refer to a study in which participants are randomly (*i.e.*, by chance) assigned to one of two or more treatment arms of a clinical trial.

831. **Range**
Refer to the difference between the smallest and largest values of a set of measurements.

832. **Rationale**
Refer to the scientific basis or hypothesis of a clinical trial.

833. **Raw Data**
Refer to all information in original records and certified copies of original records of clinical findings, observations, or other activities in a clinical trial necessary for the reconstruction and evaluation of the trial. Source data are contained in source documents.

834. Records Retention
Refer to the length of time for which trial records should be retained as per the stipulated guidelines.

835. Recruitment
Refer to the act of enrolling subjects with the proper inclusion criteria.

836. Recruitment Period
Refer to the time period for completing the recruitment of all subjects in a study.

837. Recruitment Target
Refer to the total number of subjects to be enrolled in a clinical trial with a further break-up on the basis of individual investigator sites.

838. Rectification Analysis
Refer to the process of identifying the root cause for a deviation/violation and the preventive measures taken to avoid it from happening again.

839. References
Refer to a list of relevant published literature on a topic along with complete citation.

840. Registered Nurse
Refer to a qualified nurse registered with the applicable regulatory authority to practice nursing.

841. Registered Pharmacist
Refer to a qualified pharmacist registered with the applicable regulatory authority to prepare and dispense drugs.

842. Registration Trial
Refer to a Phase-III clinical trial intended to obtain marketing authorization for a drug product under investigations.

843. Regulation
Refer to a governmental order with the force of the law.

844. Regulatory Affairs
Refer to the job function that deals with regulatory authorities.

845. Regulatory Agencies
Refer to the drug authorities or Food and Drug Administrations that have authority to regulate.

846. Regulatory Approval
Refer to permission of regulatory agencies to undertake a clinical trial or market a drug.

847. Regulatory Authorities
Same as Regulatory Agencies.

848. Regulatory Compliance
Refer to the act of following applicable regulations while undertaking an activity.

849. **Regulatory Inspections**
Refer to the act of reviewing documents, facilities, records and any other resources by a regulatory authority at a trial site or the sponsor's and/or contract research organization's facilities or at other establishment deemed appropriate by the regulatory authority.

850. **Regulatory Letter**
Refer to a letter issued by a regulatory authority summarizing the observations of regulatory inspections and the actions required thereon.

851. **Rehabilitation**
Refer to a treatment designed to facilitate the process of recovery from injury, illness or disease to as normal condition as possible.

852. **Related Event**
Refer to an adverse event that is related to the administration of investigational product.

853. **Relatedness**
Refer to the extent of relation between occurrence of an adverse event and administration of a drug/placebo.

854. **Relevant History**
Refer to a clinical history that is relevant to a particular condition or occurrence of an adverse event.

855. **Remission**
Refer to the regression of a disease condition.

856. **Remote Data Entry**
Refer to entry in the electronic case report form using a computer and modem through a distant location.

857. **Remuneration**
Payment to the study subjects for participation in a clinical trial.

858. **Reporting Database**
Refer to the database use to run the statistical reports/outputs.

859. **Representative**
Refer to an individual or juridical or other body authorized under applicable law to consent for the subject's participation in a clinical trial on behalf of a prospective subject.

860. **Reproductive Studies**
A type of toxicological testing (up to 9 months) in 2 species of animals to determine the effects of drug on fertility and reproduction and expose any teratogenic effects.

861. **Research**
Refer to systematic investigation designed to develop new/innovative products, processes or services as well as improvisation of the existing products, processes or services.

862. **Research and Development**
Refer to a department or function that is involved in discovering new/innovative products, processes or services as well as improvisation in the existing products, processes or services.

863. **Research Assistant**
Refer to a person who assists the Investigator in the conduct of research project.

864. **Research Associate**
Refer to a person who monitors the research project in order to ensure compliance with the protocol and applicable regulatory guidelines.

865. **Research Coordinator**
Same as Research Assistant.

866. **Research Ethics Board**
An independent body (a review board or a committee) constituted of medical professionals and non-medical members whose responsibility is to ensure the protection of the rights, safety and well being of human subjects involved in a clinical trial and to provide public assurance of that protection by, among other things, reviewing and approving/providing favorable opinion on, the trial protocol, the suitability of the investigator(s), facilities, and the methods and material to be used in obtaining and documenting informed consent of the trial subjects.

867. **Research Hypothesis**
Refer to the scientific rationale behind a research project.

868. **Research Misconduct**
Refer to willful misconduct (such as falsification of data) in the conduct of a research project.

869. **Research Nurse**
Refer to a qualified nurse who assists the investigator in the conduct of research project.

870. **Research Projects**
Refer to systematic investigation designed to develop new/innovative products, processes or services as well as improvisation of the existing products, processes or services.

871. **Research Protocol**
A document that describes the objective(s), design, methodology, statistical considerations and organization of a trial. The protocol also gives the background rationale for the trial.

872. **Research Record**
All information in original records of clinical findings, observations or other activities in a clinical trial necessary for the reconstruction and evaluation of the trial.

873. **Research Subject**
Refer to an individual who participates in a clinical trial or a BA/BE study.

874. Research Team

A research team includes representatives of Sponsor, CRO and Investigator site. At a clinical trial site it includes investigator, sub investigator and clinical research coordinator involved with the study.

875. Respect for Persons

Refer to an ethical principle having two separate moral requirements: (1) the requirement to acknowledge autonomy of an individual and (2) the requirement to protect those individuals with diminished autonomy.

876. Respite Care

Refer to temporary or periodic care provided in a nursing home or a healthcare centre so that the usual caregiver can take rest.

877. Responder

Refer to a subject who demonstrates response to the treatment under investigation in a clinical trial.

878. Restraints

Refer to a condition of being restrained.

879. Retrospective Study

Refer to a study that is based on historical data already existing in the records.

880. Review of Research

Refer to ethical, scientific and medical review of a research proposal by an ethics committee.

881. Revision

Refer to an amendment in the existing documents or processes.

882. Revision Summary

Refer to a point-wise summary of additions and/or deletions made to an existing document or process.

883. Risk

Refer to a factor, element or course of action involving an uncertain, potentially negative outcome.

884. Risk Benefit Analysis

Refer to an analysis of potential benefit of a clinical trial along with the associated risk.

885. Risk Benefit Balance

Refer to risk to individual subject *vs.* potential benefits.

886. Risk Benefit Ratio

Same as Risk Benefit Balance.

887. Roles and Responsibilities

Refer to delegation of specific duties to trial personnel.

888. **Root Cause**

Refer to the causative factor for a deviation or event.

889. **Route of Administration**

Refer to the system of drug delivery to the human body (*e.g.* oral, injectable, local *etc.*).

890. **Routine Monitoring**

Refer to the act of overseeing the progress of a clinical trial and of ensuring that it is conducted, recorded, and reported in accordance with the Protocol, Standard Operating Procedures (SOPs), Good Clinical Practice (GCP) and the applicable regulatory requirements.

S

891. **Safety**
Refer to the absence of adverse event from a drug product.

892. **Safety Assessment**
Refer to the assessment of adverse events and serious adverse events experienced by the participants in a clinical trial.

893. **Safety Reports**
Report prepared from a serious and unexpected adverse experience.

894. **Sample Size**
The number of patients required to achieve the desired statistical significance in a clinical trial.

895. **Sampling Plan**
Refer to a plan that highlights the specific description of the data to be collected.

896. **Scatter Plots**
These displays relation between two numeric variables while distinguishing between levels of categorical variables.

897. **Scheduled Continuation Review**
Refer to the ongoing periodic review of trial progress by the ethics committee.

898. **Scientific Misconduct**
Refer to willful non-compliance such as lack of supervision or falsification of data.

899. **Screening Log**
Refer to a log that captures the details of all the subjects screened for a clinical trial.

900. **Screening Trials**
Refer to trials which test the best way to detect certain diseases or health conditions.

901. **Script**
Refer to a sequence of instructions that are interpreted or carried out by another program.

902. **Sequential Analysis**
A type of statistical analysis where the sample size is not fixed in advance. In sequential analysis data is evaluated as it is collected and further sampling is stopped in accordance with a pre-defined stopping rule as soon as significant results are observed.

903. **Sequential Design**
A trial design that looks at the data at a particular time points or after a defined number of subjects have been entered and followed up based on formulating a stopping rule

derived from repeated significance tests.

904. **Serendipity**
Refer to discovery by chance.

905. **Serious Adverse Drug Experience**
Any untoward medical occurrence that at any dose: results in death, is life-threatening, requires inpatient hospitalization or prolongation of existing hospitalization, results in persistent or significant disability/incapacity, results in a congenital anomaly/birth defect.

906. **Serious Adverse Drug Reaction**
Same as Serious Adverse Drug Experience.

907. **Serious Adverse Event**
Same as Serious Adverse Drug Experience.

908. **Seriousness Criteria**
Refer to criteria that classify an adverse event as serious adverse events such as: results in death, is life-threatening, requires inpatient hospitalization or prolongation of existing hospitalization, results in persistent or significant disability/incapacity, results in a congenital anomaly/birth defect.

909. **Server**
Refer to a computer that acts as a gateway for providing one or more services over a computer network.

910. **Severe Adverse Event**
Refer to the severity of an adverse event that causes significant discomfort to a subject and requires treatment on an urgent basis.

911. **Severity**
Refer to the intensity of an adverse event.

912. **Shipment/Inventory Forms**
Refer to the document(s) that are sent along with a shipment and contains a complete description of the product (*e.g.* strength, quantity, supplier's details *etc.*) being shipped.

913. **Side Effect**
Refer to any untoward medical occurrence in a patient or clinical investigation subject who have been administered a pharmaceutical product and that does not necessarily have a causal relationship with the product.

914. **Significant**
Refer to the power or strength of the results of an intervention *vis-à-vis* comparator.

915. **Signs**
Refer to the physical abnormalities that are linked to an adverse event.

916. **Single Blind Study**
Refer to a study in which the subject is unaware of which medication he/she is taking.

917. Single Center Study
Refer to a clinical trial which is conducted at one trial site only.

918. Single Masked
Same as Single Blind Study.

919. Site
Refer to a facility where clinical trials are conducted.

920. Site Assessment
Refer to a systematic review of investigator's qualification, facility, infrastructure, patient load *etc.* by a Sponsor's representative in order to select the sites for conducting a clinical trial.

921. Site Assessment Visit Report
Refer to a written report prepared by Sponsor's representative that summarizes the observations and findings of site assessment visit.

922. Site Audit
Refer to a systematic and independent examination of trial related activities and documents at a trial site to determine whether the evaluated trial related activities were conducted and the data were recorded, analyzed and accurately reported according to the protocol, sponsor's Standard Operating Procedures (SOPs), Good Clinical Practice (GCP), and the applicable regulatory requirement(s).

923. Site Closeout
Refer to the activity of closing the trial sites at the end of study or at study termination after all the requirements have been fulfilled.

924. Site Closure
Same as Site Closeout.

925. Site Code
Refer to the unique number assigned to individual trial site for its identification.

926. Site Contact List
Refer to a list that contains the names and contact details of all the participating sites in a trial.

927. Site Coordinator
Refer to a person employed at clinical investigator's site to record the clinical trial data in compliance with protocol, GCP and applicable regulatory guidelines.

928. Site Delegation Log
A document that enlists the specific trial related duties performed by individual study team members along with their signatures and/or initials.

929. Site Evaluation Report
Refer to a written report prepared by Sponsor's representative that summarizes the observations and findings of site assessment visit.

930. **Site Identification List**
Refer to a list that contains the names and contact details of all the participating sites in a trial.

931. **Site Initiation**
Refer to the activation of a site for initiating a clinical trial after the ethics committee and regulatory approval has been obtained and other trial specific requirements have been fulfilled.

932. **Site Management**
Refer to the act of coordinating and managing a trial at a site.

933. **Site Management Organization (SMO)**
Organization responsible for managing the investigator sites (by appointing a study coordinator) in a clinical trial.

934. **Site Master File**
Refer to a file that contains all the essential trial documents at a trial site.

935. **Site Qualification Visit Report**
Same as Site Evaluation Report.

936. **Site Selection Report**
Same as Site Evaluation Report.

937. **Site Training**
Refer to imparting training to site personnel on study protocol, GCP and applicable regulatory processes.

938. **Site Visit Log**
Refer to a log that captures the details of visit made by Sponsor/CRO's representative at a trial site.

939. **Skilled Care**
Refer to a type of health care given when skilled nursing or rehabilitation staff is required to manage, observe, and evaluate the care.

940. **Skilled Nursing Care**
Refer to a level of health care that can only be performed safely and correctly by a licensed nurse.

941. **Social Worker**
Refer to a person that provides social services.

942. **Source Data**
All information in original records (and certified copies of original records) of clinical findings, observations or other activities in a clinical trial necessary for the reconstruction and evaluation of the trial. Source data are contained in source documents.

943. **Source Data/Document Verification**
Refer to the verification of source documents and other trial records for accuracy,

completion and compliance with protocol, GCP and applicable regulatory guidelines.

944. **Source Documents**
Original documents, data, and records (*e.g.* hospital records, clinical and office charts, laboratory notes, memoranda, subjects' diaries or evaluation checklists, pharmacy dispensing records, recorded data from automated instruments, copies or transcriptions certified after verification as being accurate copies, microfiches, photographic negatives, microfilm or magnetic media, X-rays, subject files, and records kept at the pharmacy, at the laboratories and at medico-technical departments involved in the clinical trial).

945. **Specialist**
Refer to a person who specializes in a particular field (*e.g.* cardiologist, oncologist, auditor *etc.*).

946. **Sponsor**
An individual, company, institution, or organization which takes responsibility for the initiation, management and/or financing of a clinical trial.

947. **Sponsor Investigator**
Refer to an individual who both initiate and conducts alone or with others a clinical trial and under whose immediate direction the investigational product is administered to, dispensed to, or used by a subject. The obligations of a sponsor-investigator include both those of a sponsor and those of an investigator.

948. **Sponsor Master File**
Refer to a file that contains all the essential trial documents at sponsor's facility.

949. **Stability**
Refer to the time period and storage condition under which a drug is stable.

950. **Stability Data**
Refer to the data on the stability of a drug product under routine and accelerated stability conditions.

951. **Staff Signature Log**
Refer to a document that enlists the specific trial related duties performed by individual study team members along with their signatures and/or initials.

952. **Standard Deviation**
Indicator of the relative variability of a variable around its mean (the square root of the variance).

953. **Standard Error**
The estimated standard deviation or error of a series of measurements.

954. **Standard Operating Procedures (SOPs)**
Detailed, written instructions to achieve uniformity in the performance of a specific task/activity.

955. **Standard of Care**
Medical management of a patient based on established regimens or guidelines.

956. **Standard Treatment or Care**
Same as Standard of Care.

957. **Start-up Meeting**
Refer to the investigator meeting conducted before initiating a clinical trial and attended by all the participating investigators and respective site personnel.

958. **Statement of Investigator**
FDA form signed and dated by the investigator before initiating a Phase 1-3 trial that outlines the obligations of investigator.

959. **Statement of Work**
Refer to description of services to be provided under the scope of an Agreement.

960. **Statistical Analysis**
Refer to providing meaning to a set of data (which otherwise would be a collection of numbers and/or values) by applying an appropriate statistical method.

961. **Statistical Analysis Plan**
A written document that contains detailed information and rationale on the statistical analysis to be undertaken for a clinical trial.

962. **Statistical Errors**
Refer to errors that can occur in a clinical trial such as a situation where the effect of therapy is confounded with another factor or when the patients on trial are not sufficiently representative of the targeted patient population. The common statistical errors are Type-1 error (alpha error) and Type-2 error (beta error).

963. **Statistical Methods**
A method of analyzing or representing the statistical data.

964. **Statistical Significance**
The probability that an event or difference occurred by chance alone. In clinical trials the level of statistical significance depends on the number of participants studied and the observations made as well as the magnitude of differences observed.

965. **Statistician**
A person having knowledge and competence of statistics.

966. **Statistics**
Refer to the process of collecting, recording and summarizing data that are collected from experiments, records and surveys.

967. **Sterility**
Refer to the absence of viable contaminating microorganisms.

968. **Stochastic**
An analysis involving a random variable.

969. **Stochastic Model**
Same as Stochastic.

970. **Stratification**
A tool used during the randomization process to ensure an exact balance between the treatment arms with respect to key patient factors that are strongly related to the outcome variable.

971. **Student's t-Test**
A comparison test to determine whether the mean value of a numeric variable (or response variable) in a given population is same as that in another population. For *e.g.* a study that investigate whether the mean hemoglobin level after a fixed treatment period of Drug A is same as that of Drug B.

972. **Study Arm**
Refer to the treatment group of a clinical trial.

973. **Study Closeout**
Refer to closing a clinical study after the same has been completed or prematurely terminated/suspended.

974. **Study Closeout Visit Report**
A written report to document that all activities required for study closeout have been completed and all the essential documents are archived in appropriate files.

975. **Study Closure**
Refer to closing a clinical study after the same has been completed or prematurely terminated/suspended.

976. **Study Coordinator**
A person employed at clinical investigator's site to record the clinical trial data in compliance with protocol, GCP and applicable regulatory guidelines. The investigator delegates specific duties to a study coordinator.

977. **Study Design**
Refer to the methodology used to investigate a drug or device for its safety and/or efficacy.

978. **Study Drug**
An investigational product or marketed product (*i.e.*, active control) or placebo used in a clinical trial.

979. **Study Endpoint**
Primary or secondary outcome(s) used to judge the effectiveness of a treatment.

980. **Study Initiation Visit Report**
A report that documents the activation of a clinical study after the ethics committee and regulatory approval has been obtained and other trial specific requirements have been fulfilled.

981. **Study Materials**
Refer to a complete set of supplies (*e.g.* documents, investigational product, laboratory kits *etc.*) to be used in a clinical trial.

982. **Study Monitor**
A person employed by the Sponsor or CRO who reviews study records at trial site(s) to determine that a study is being conducted in accordance with the protocol and applicable regulatory guidelines.

983. **Study Number**
A unique identifier assigned to a clinical study for its easy identification.

984. **Study Nurse**
Refer to a qualified nurse who assists the investigator in the conduct of research project.

985. **Study Start-up Visit Report**
Same as Study Initiation Visit Report.

986. **Study Subject**
An individual who participates in a clinical trial either as a recipient of the investigational product or as a control.

987. **Study Supplies**
Refer to a complete set of supplies (*e.g.* documents, investigational product, laboratory kits *etc.*) to be used in a clinical trial.

988. **Study Team**
A group of individuals that constitutes the research team.

989. **Study Timelines**
Refer to the sequence of study related activities arranged on a time-scale.

990. **Study Treatment**
Refer to the modality of medical management of a trial patient(s).

991. **Study Type**
Refer to the type of a clinical study based on its design (*e.g.* open label, blinded, single-arm, two-arm *etc.*).

992. **Sub-investigator**
Any individual member of the clinical trial team designated and supervised by the investigator to perform trial-related procedures and/or to make important trial-related decisions (*e.g.* associates, residents, research fellows) at a site.

993. **Sub-acute Toxicity**
A type of toxicological testing of a drug in 2 species of animals that usually lasts for 6 months.

994. **Sub-contract**
A contract to perform a part of or all of the obligations of another's contract.

995. Sub-contracting
The act of executing a sub-contract.

996. Subgroup Analysis
Exploratory secondary analyses performed to gain more insight into various aspects of the trial. For *e.g.* comparison of study results in males *vs.* females participants.

997. Subject
An individual who participates in a clinical trial either as a recipient of the investigational product or as a control.

998. Subject Enrollment Log
Refer to a log that captures the dates of enrolment and other protocol required visits of a clinical trial subject.

999. Subject Identification Code
A unique identifier assigned to trial subjects for protecting their identity.

1000. Subject Identification Code List
A confidential list maintained by a trial site that captures names of all the trial subjects *vis-à-vis* their allocated subject number/code.

1001. Subject Identification List
Same as Subject Identification Code List.

1002. Subject Number
Same as Subject Identification Code.

1003. Supersede
Refer to replacing a document with the new one after the same has been revised/updated.

1004. Supervisor
A person with the authority to oversee the work of a person or group.

1005. Surrogate Endpoints
Physiological or biochemical markers that can be measured quickly and easily and that are taken as being predictive of important clinical outcomes.

1006. Survival Analysis
The analysis of survival data.

1007. Survival Data
Refer to any time-to-event variable. In clinical trials, common example of survival data includes: time to response, time to relapse, time in remission, time to discontinuation *etc.*

1008. Survivor Function
The probability that an individual will survive up to at least a certain time. The estimate for the survivor function is called as **Kaplan-Meier** estimate.

21

T

1009. Target Selection
A drug discovery approach that involves choosing a disease or biological target (such as enzyme, receptor, ion channel *etc.*) to treat and then developing a model for that disease.

1010. Telephone Log
A list/log that captures the details of telephonic discussion in a clinical trial.

1011. Temperature logs
A log that captures the storage temperature (minimum/maximum) of investigational product on a daily basis.

1012. Template
A pre-designed form/document that include standard fill-in-the-blanks spaces for capturing the standard information.

1013. Teratogenic
Refer to substances or agents that can interfere with normal embryonic development.

1014. Termination of the Study
Pre-mature suspension of a clinical study due to lack of efficacy or safety or funding.

1015. Therapeutic Window
The concentration range over which a drug has a therapeutic effect without having unacceptable toxicity.

1016. Third Party Outsourcing
The act of sub-contracting a part of or all of the obligations of a contract to a third party not included in the initial contract.

1017. Toxicity
An adverse effect produced by a drug that is detrimental to the participant's health.

1018. Toxicology Testing
Studies (carried out both *in-vitro* and on animal species) to determine the potential risk of a compound to man and the environment.

1019. Trademark
A name, word, symbol or phrases used to identify a particular product.

1020. Training Log
A documented trail of all the trainings undertaken by clinical research personnel. It generally includes the topic of the training, training modality, completion date and signature of the personnel.

1021. Training Records
Same as Training Log.

1022. Translation

The act of transforming document, text or phrases from one language to another language.

1023. Treatment IND

A type of non-commercial Investigational New Drug Application whereby Food and Drug Administration can permit an investigational drug to be used while the final clinical work and review is still ongoing, if there is preliminary evidence of drug efficacy and the drug is intended to treat a serious or life-threatening disease, or if there is no comparable alternative drug or therapy available to treat that stage of disease in the intended patient population.

1024. Trelis Plots

Graphical display of relationship between variables (across the levels of multiple categorical variables). These are useful for investigating the need of sub-group analysis.

1025. Trial Arm

Refer to the treatment group of a clinical trial.

1026. Trial Audit

A systematic and independent examination of trial related activities and documents to determine whether the evaluated trial related activities were conducted and the data were recorded, analyzed and accurately reported according to the protocol, sponsor's Standard Operating Procedures (SOPs), Good Clinical Practice (GCP), and the applicable regulatory requirement(s).

1027. Trial Master File (TMF)

A central file in which all the essential clinical trial documents are filed.

1028. Trial Number

A unique identifier assigned to a clinical study for its easy identification.

1029. Trial Site

The location or facility where a clinical trial is conducted.

1030. Trial Subject

An individual who participates in a clinical trial either as a recipient of the investigational product or as a control.

1031. Trial Suspension

Pre-mature termination of a clinical trial due to lack of efficacy or safety or funding.

1032. Triple Blind

A study design in which the knowledge of treatment assignment is concealed from the personnel who organize and analyze the data as well as from the investigators and study subjects.

1033. Two-stage Design

A study design in which response rate is assessed after a predetermined number of patients have been observed and the study is either terminated or allowed to continue depending on the outcome.

U

1034. Unblinding
The act of breaking the blinding codes of a clinical trial.

1035. Uncontrolled Clinical Trial
A trial design that does not contain a control arm.

1036. Unexpected Adverse Drug Reaction
An adverse reaction, the nature or severity of which is not consistent with the applicable product information (*e.g.* Investigator's Brochure for an unapproved investigational product or package insert/summary of product characteristics for an approved product).

1037. Unplanned Analysis
A situation where the trial data is analyzed at a time-point which is not specified in the protocol or statistical analysis plan.

V

1038. Validation Certificate
A document to demonstrate that a procedure, process and activity will consistently lead to the expected results.

1039. Vendor
Refer to a supplier of goods or services.

1040. Vernacular Language
Refer to the native language of a country or a place.

1041. Version
Refer to the number assigned to an essential document in use. Version number is important to provide an audit trail.

1042. Version Control
The act of assigning the version number to an essential clinical trial document.

1043. Visitor's Log
A log that captures the details of personnel (such as date of visit, purpose of visit *etc.*) who visits a clinical trial site.

1044. Voluntary
The act of giving one's own free will without any coercion or undue inducement.

1045. Voluntary Action Indicated
A classification of regulatory inspection outcome that requires voluntary action or response.

1046. Volunteer
An individual who voluntarily participates in a clinical trial either as a recipient of the investigational product or as a control.

1047. Voting Members
Refer to the ethics committee members who participate in a meeting and provide their opinion on a clinical trial proposal.

1048. Vulnerable Populations
Individuals whose willingness to volunteer in a clinical trial may be unduly influenced by the expectation, whether justified or not, of benefits associated with participation or of a retaliatory response from senior members of a hierarchy in case of refusal to participate. Examples are members of a group with a hierarchical structure (medical, pharmacy, dental and nursing students), subordinate hospital and laboratory personnel, employees of the pharmaceutical industry, members of the armed forces, and persons kept in detention. Other vulnerable subjects include patients with

incurable diseases, persons in nursing homes, unemployed or impoverished persons, patients in emergency situations, ethnic minority groups, homeless persons, nomads, refugees, minors and those incapable of giving consent.

1049. Vulnerable Subjects
Same as Vulnerable Populations.

24

W

1050. Well-being

A state of physical and mental soundness.

1051. Wilcoxin Rank Sum Test

A statistical test to determine whether two population groups have the same value of a response variable. This test requires the presence of two comparison groups. For *e.g.* a study that investigate frequency of a specific adverse event between two groups of patients.

1052. Wilcoxon Signed Rank Test

A non-parametric equivalent of the paired t-test. This test requires 1 population group with 2 measurements of numeric variable per patient. For *e.g.* a study that investigate within-group change from baseline to endpoint of a given numeric variable, where the change variable does not follow a normal distribution.

Abbreviations

Sl. No.	Abbreviation	Description
1	AADA	Abbreviated Antibiotic Drug Application
2	ABPI	Association of the British Pharmaceutical Industry
3	ACDM	Association of Clinical Data Management
4	ADR	Adverse Drug Reaction
5	AE	Adverse Event
6	ANDA	Abbreviated New Drug Application
7	ANOVA	Analysis of Variance
8	AQL	Acceptable Quality Level
9	BA	Bioavailability
10	BE	Bioequivalence
11	BIMO	Bioresearch Monitoring
12	BLA	Biologics License Application
13	BP	British Pharmacopoeia
14	BPR	Batch Production Records
15	BSA	Body Surface Area
16	CBER	Center for Biologics Evaluation and Research
17	CDA	Confidentiality Disclosure Agreement
18	CDC	Clinical Data Coordinator
19	CDER	Center for Drug Evaluation and Research
20	CDISC	Clinical Data Interchange Standards Consortium
21	CDM	Clinical Data Management
22	CDM	Clinical Data Manager
23	CDS	Clinical Data Specialist
24	CDSCO	Central Drug Standard Control Organization
25	CEC	Clinical Endpoint Committee
26	CFR	Code of Federal Regulations
27	CI	Chief Investigator
28	CI	Co-Investigator

Sl. No.	Abbreviation	Description
29	CIB	Clinical Investigator Brochure
30	CIOMS	Council for International Organizations of Medical Sciences
31	CME	Continuing Medical Education
32	COA	Certificate of Analysis
33	COREC	Central Office for Research Ethics Committees
34	COSTART	Coding Symbols for a Thesaurus of Adverse Reaction Terms
35	CPMP	Committee for Proprietary Medicinal Products
36	CRA	Clinical Research Associate/Clinical Research Assistant
37	CRC	Clinical Research Coordinator
38	CRF	Case Report Form
39	CRO	Contract Research Organization
40	CSM	Committee on Safety of Medicines
41	CSR	Clinical Study Report
42	CSVP	Computer System Validation Plan
43	CT	Clinical Trial
44	CTA	Clinical Trial Administrator
45	CTA	Clinical Trial Application/Authorization
46	CTA	Clinical Trial Agreement
47	CTC	Clinical Trial Coordinator
48	CTD	Common Technical Document
49	CTN	Clinical Trial Notification
50	CTNR	Clinical Trials Not for Registration
51	CTM	Clinical Trials Monitor
52	CTSU	Cancer Trials Support Unit
53	CTSU	Clinical Trials Service Unit
54	CTX	Clinical Trials Exemption
55	CV	Curriculum Vitae
56	DBL	Database Lock
57	DBMS	Database Management System
58	DBQR	Database Quality Review
59	DCGI	Drug Controller General of India
60	DCC	Drugs Consultative Committee

Sl. No.	Abbreviation	Description
61	DCF	Data Clarification Form
62	DDE	Dynamic Data Exchange
63	DDX	Doctors and Dentists Exemption
64	DFS	Disease Free Survival
65	DGFT	Directorate General of Foreign Trade
66	DHHS	Department of Health and Human Services
67	DM	Data Manager
68	DM	Data Management
69	DMC	Data Management Center
70	DMC	Data Management Coordinator
71	DMF	Drug Master File
72	DNDE	Data Not for Data Entry
73	DOB	Date of Birth
74	DOD	Date of Death
75	DQF	Data Query Form
76	DSMB	Data Safety Monitoring Board
77	DSMC	Data Safety Monitoring Committee
78	DSMP	Data Safety Monitoring Plan
79	DTAB	Drugs Technical Advisory Board
80	DVP	Data Validation Plan
81	E3	Structure and Content of Clinical Study Report
82	E6	Good Clinical Practice: Consolidated Guidance
83	E9	Statistical Principles for Clinical Trials
84	EC	Ethics Committee
85	e-CRF	Electronic Case Report Form
86	EDC	Electronic Data Capture
87	EDD	Early Drug Development
88	EFPIA	European Federation of Pharmaceutical Industries and Associations
89	EIR	Establishment Inspection Report
90	EU	European Union
91	EMEA	European Agency for the Evaluation of Medicinal Products
92	EPA	Environmental Protection Agency

Sl. No.	Abbreviation	Description
93	ER	Electronic Records
94	ERB	Ethics Review Board
95	ES	Electronic Signature
96	EU	European Union
97	FDA	Food and Drug Administration (US)
98	FDF	Financial Disclosure Form
99	FED	Field Edit Description
100	FIA	Freedom of Information Act
101	FOI	Freedom of Information
102	FPV	First Patient Visit
103	FSR	Final Study Report
104	FTP	File Transfer Protocol
105	GC	Gas Chromatography
106	GCP	Good Clinical Practice
107	GDP	Good Documentation Practice
108	GEAC	Genetic Engineering Approval Committee
109	INN	International Nonproprietary Names
110	IP	Indian Pharmacopoeia
111	GLP	Good Laboratory Practice
112	GMP	Good Manufacturing Practice
113	HE	Health Economics
114	HHS	Health and Human Services
115	HIPAA	Health Insurance Portability and Accountability Act
116	HPLC	High Performance Liquid Chromatography
117	HTML	Hypertext Markup Language
118	HTS	High Throughput Screening
119	IB	Investigator's Brochure
120	ICD	Informed Consent Document
121	ICD	International Classification of Diseases
122	ICF	Informed Consent Form
123	ICH	International Conference on Harmonisation
124	ICMR	Indian Council of Medical Research

Sl. No.	Abbreviation	Description
125	IDE	Investigational Device Exemption
126	IDMC	Independent Data Monitoring Committee
127	IDSMB	Independent Data and Safety Monitoring Board
128	IEC	Independent Ethics Committee/Institutional Ethics Committee
129	IEC	Import Export Code
130	IFPMA	International Federation of Pharmaceutical Manufactures Association
131	IIT	Investigator Initiated Trial
132	IM	Investigator Meeting
133	IMF	Investigator Master File
134	IMP	Investigational Medicinal Product
135	IND	Investigational New Drug
136	IP	Investigational Product
137	IRB	Institutional Review Board
138	ISM	Investigator Safety Mailings
139	IT	Information Technology
140	IU	Investigator's Undertaking
141	IVRS	Interactive Voice Response System
142	KPI	Key Performance Indicators
143	LAN	Local Area Network
144	LAR	Legally Acceptable Representative
145	LFU	Lost to Follow-up
146	LOA	Letter of Agreement
147	LOC	Letter of Confidentiality
148	LOI	Letter of Intent
149	LPV	Last Patient Visit
150	MAH	Marketing Authorization Holder
151	MCA	Medicines Control Agency
152	MEC	Minimum Effective Concentration
153	MedDRA	Medical Dictionary for Regulatory Activities
154	MHRA	Medicines and Healthcare Products Regulatory Authority
155	MOA	Mechanism of Action/Mode of Administration
156	MOU	Memorandum of Understanding

Sl. No.	Abbreviation	Description
157	MRC	Medical Research Council
158	MRC	Medical Registration Certificate
159	MSA	Master Service Agreement
160	MTD	Maximum Tolerated Dose
161	NAI	No Action Indicated
162	NCE	New Chemical Entity
163	NCI	National Cancer Institute
164	NCR	No Carbon Required
165	NDA	Non Disclosure Agreement
166	NDA	New Drug Application
167	NF	National Formulary
168	NGO	Non Governmental Organization
169	NHS	National Health Service
170	OAI	Official Action Indicated
171	ODM	Operational Data Model
172	OHRP	Office for Human Research Protection
173	OR	Odds Ratio
174	OS	Overall Survival
175	OTC	Over The Counter
176	PDF	Portable Document Format
177	PHI	Protected Health Information
178	PHI	Personal Health Identifier
179	PI	Principal Investigator
180	PMS	Post Marketing Surveillance/Post Marketing Studies
181	PRC	Protocol Review Committee
182	PS	Performance Status
183	PSA	Professional Services Agreement
184	PSUR	Periodic Safety Update Report
185	QA	Quality Assurance
186	QAA	Quality Assurance Administrator
187	QAM	Quality Assurance Manager
188	QC	Quality Control

Sl. No.	Abbreviation	Description
189	QOL	Quality of Life
190	QLQ	Quality of Life Questionnaire
191	RCT	Randomized Control Trial
192	R&D	Research and Development
193	RDE	Remote Data Entry
194	SAE	Serious Adverse Event
195	SAP	Statistical Analysis Plan
196	SAR	Serious Adverse Reaction/ Structure Activity Relationship
197	SAS	Statistical Analytical System
198	SC	Steering Committee
199	SDMB	Safety Data Monitoring Boards
200	SDTM	Study Data Tabulation Model
201	SDV	Source Data Verification
202	SI	Sub-Investigator
203	SIV	Site Initiation Visit
204	SMF	Site Master File
205	SMO	Site Management Organization
206	SOP	Standard Operating Procedure
207	SPC	Summary of Product Characteristics
208	SQL	Structured Query Language
209	SSAR	Suspected Serious Adverse Reaction
210	SUSAR	Suspected Unexpected Serious Adverse Reaction
211	TAG	Trial Advisory Group
212	TGA	Therapeutics Goods Administration
213	TESS	Treatment Emergent Signs and Symptoms
214	TLF	Tables, Listings and Figures
215	TLG	Tables, Listings and Graphs
216	TMF	Trial Master File
217	TMG	Trial Management Group
218	ULN	Upper Laboratory Normal
219	USP	United State Pharmacopoeia
220	VAI	Voluntary Action Indicated

Sl. No.	Abbreviation	Description
221	WAN	Wide Area Network
222	WHO	World Health Organization
223	WMA	World Medical Association
224	WNL	With in Normal Limits

26

Clinical Trial Stakeholders

Clinical Research is a team effort and requires involvement of various stakeholders to achieve the planned endpoint. Each stakeholder has a defined role and success can not be accomplished without involving individual stakeholder.

The various stakeholders include:

- Sponsor/ Contract Research Organization (CRO)
- Investigator
- Ethics Committee (EC)
- Regulatory Authority (*e.g.* FDA in US, DCGI in India *etc.*)
- Patients/Study Subjects

Sponsor/CRO

Sponsor refers to an individual, company, institution, or organization which takes responsibility for the initiation, management, and/or financing of a clinical trial.

Contract Research Organization (CRO) refers to a person or an organization (commercial, academic, or other) contracted by the sponsor to perform one or more of a sponsor's trial-related duties and functions.

The chief responsibilities of Sponsor/CRO are:
- Trial planning, development of essential trial documents and allocation of resources
- Logistics planning and appointment of central lab, CRO and other vendors
- Manufacturing and accountability of investigational product
- Investigator's selection and site set-up
- Regulatory submission and obtaining trial approval, import/export licenses
- Conducting investigator's training meeting
- Clinical trial monitoring
- Data management
- Pharmacovigilance
- Ensuring compliance with protocol, GCP and applicable regulatory guidelines
- Clinical trial auditing/quality assurance
- Preparation of clinical study report
- Trial closure
- Publication of trial results
- Obtaining marketing approval

Investigator

Investigator refers to a person who is responsible for the conduct of a clinical trial at a site.

The chief responsibilities of a clinical trial investigator are:
- Site organization and constitution of study team
- Delegation of responsibilities at site

> Submission of trial document to ethics committee and obtaining approval
> Trial initiation at site
> Administration of informed consent to study subjects
> Medical care of study subjects
> Source data documentation
> Medical record maintenance
> Drug dispensing and accountability
> Ensuring compliance with protocol, GCP and applicable regulatory guidelines
> Management of adverse events
> Reporting of serious adverse events to sponsor and ethics committee
> Communication with ethics committee and sponsor/CRO
> Site closure

Ethics Committee

Ethics committee refers to an independent body, constituted of medical professionals and non-medical members, whose responsibility is to ensure the protection of the rights, safety and well being of human subjects involved in a clinical trial and to provide public assurance of that protection by among other things, reviewing and approving/providing favorable opinion on, the trial protocol, the suitability of the investigator(s), facilities, and the methods and material to be used in obtaining and documenting informed consent of the trial subjects. Ethics committee is also called as Institutional Review Board (IRB), Institutional Ethics Committee (IEC) and Ethics Review Board (ERB).

The chief responsibilities of Ethics Committee are:
> Constitution and organization of ethics committee
> Review and approval of trial documents
> Meeting 'quorum' requirements
> Maintaining minutes of ethics meetings
> Review of protocol violations, adverse events/serious adverse events and periodic reports
> Ensuring compliance with GCP and applicable regulatory guidelines

Regulatory Authority

Regulatory authority refers to the drug control authorities or Food and Drug Administrations that have the authority to regulate.

The chief responsibilities of Regulatory Authority are:
> Laying down the rules and regulations
> Review of trial documents and granting trial permission/approval
> Review of protocol violations, adverse events/serious adverse events and periodic reports
> Termination/suspension of trial (if deemed appropriate)
> Inspection (Sponsor, CRO, Investigator, IRB/EC/IEC etc.)

Study Subject

Study subject refers to an individual who participates in a clinical trial.

The chief responsibilities of Study subject are:
> Voluntary consent for participation in a clinical trial
> Compliance with protocol schedule of events

Clinical Study Process

27

Clinical Study Process Part- 1: Initiating a Clinical Trial

Project Feasibility Assessment and Study Milestones Planning
(by Sponsor)

↓

Constitution of Core Study Team (by Sponsor)

↓

Development of Essential Trial Documents (by Sponsor)
(protocol, IB, ICD, CRF, data management guidelines/systems)

↓

Financial Planning and Grants Allocation (by Sponsor)

↓

Selection of CROs/Central Lab/Data Management Center etc.
(by Sponsor)

↓

Investigational Agent Co-ordination (by Sponsor)
(inventory planning, manufacturing, handling and storage)

↓

Site Selection (by Sponsor)

↓

Contracts and Agreements (by Sponsor and Investigator)

↓

Preparation of Trial Binders (by Sponsor)
(project file, investigator site file, training binders, lab manuals etc.)

↓

Translations of ICD and relevant documents in regional languages
(by Sponsor)

↓

Regulatory Submission (by Sponsor)

↓

↓

Regulatory Approvals (by Regulatory Authority)

↓

Ethics Committee (EC) Submission (by Investigator)

↓

EC Approval (by Ethics Committee)

↓

Investigator Site Training (by Sponsor)

↓

Study Initiation (by Sponsor)

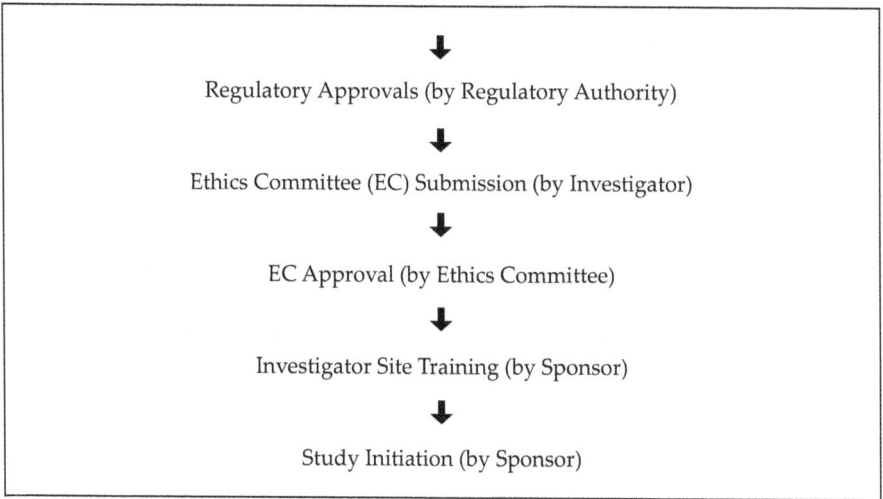

* Sponsor may designate any or all of its responsibilities to a CRO

Clinical Study Process Part- 2: Conduct of a Clinical Trial

Study Initiation (by Sponsor)

↓

Trial Conduct (by Investigator)
(recruitment of study subjects, delegation of duties at the site,
administration of ICD, administration of investigational
product/comparator, medical care of study subjects, data collection and
management, management and reporting of AEs/SAEs, compliance
with protocol schedule of events, compliance with ICG-GCP and
applicable regulatory guidelines)

↓

Participation in the Trial (by Patient/Study Subject)
(voluntary consent, compliance with protocol schedule of events)

↓

Monitoring of Trial (by Sponsor)
(Checking of protocol compliance, drug accountability, GCP
compliance, audit trail, data collection, regulatory compliance, good
documentation)

↓

Overall Site Management (by Investigator)

↓

Management of Logistics and Clinical Trial Supplies (by Sponsor)

↓

Adverse Events Recording and Reporting (by Investigator)

↓

Ongoing Data Management (by Sponsor)

↓

Periodic Reporting to Ethics Committee (by Investigator)

↓

Periodic Reporting to Regulatory Agencies (by Sponsor)

↓

⬇

Meeting the Project Timelines (by Sponsor and Investigator)

⬇

Payments as per Schedule (by Sponsor)

⬇

Amendment(s) to the Study, if required (by Sponsor)

⬇

Quality Assurance (by Sponsor)

⬇

Ongoing Training and Development for new/existing staff (by Sponsor)

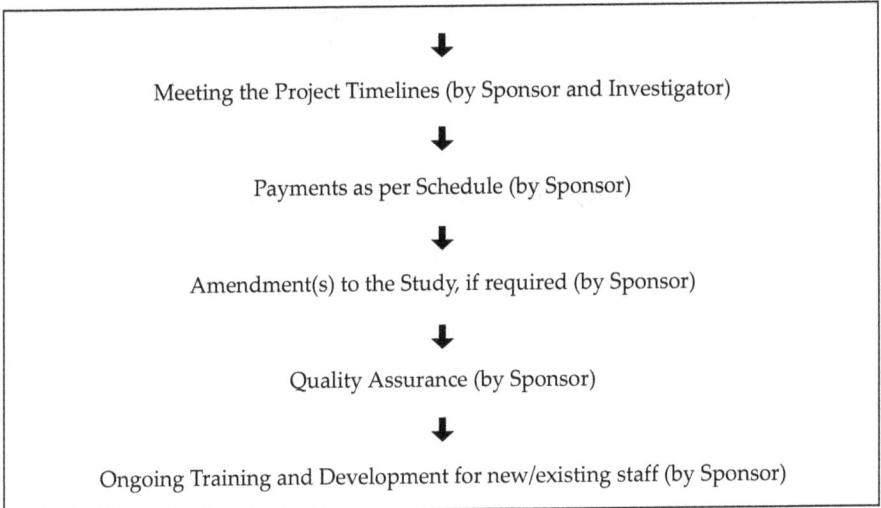

* Sponsor may designate any or all of its responsibilities to a CRO

Clinical Study Process Part- 3: Closure of a Clinical Trial

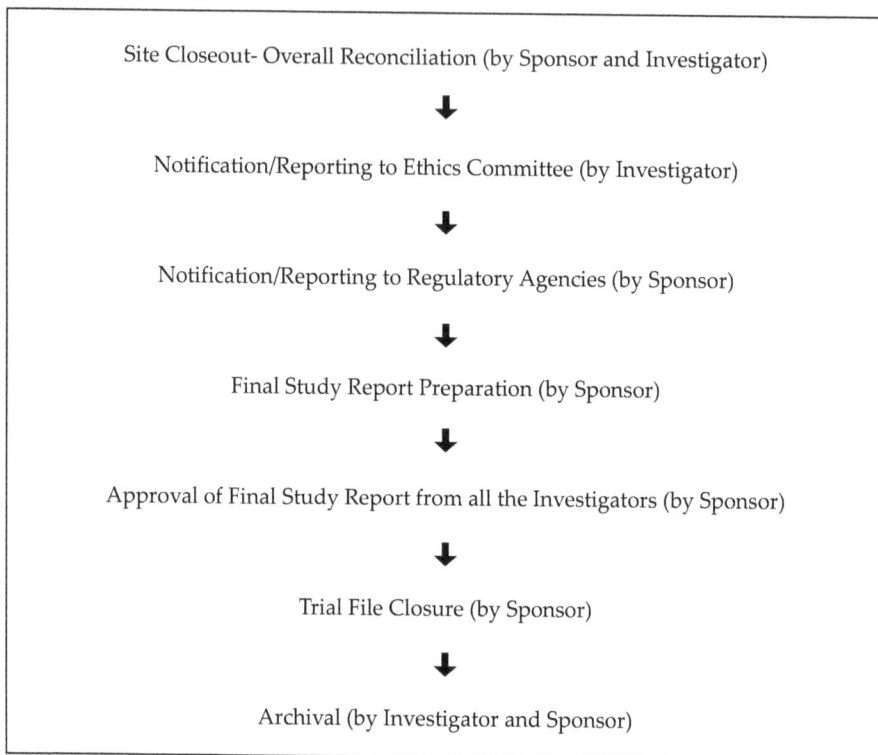

Site Closeout- Overall Reconciliation (by Sponsor and Investigator)

↓

Notification/Reporting to Ethics Committee (by Investigator)

↓

Notification/Reporting to Regulatory Agencies (by Sponsor)

↓

Final Study Report Preparation (by Sponsor)

↓

Approval of Final Study Report from all the Investigators (by Sponsor)

↓

Trial File Closure (by Sponsor)

↓

Archival (by Investigator and Sponsor)

Clinical Study Process Part- 4: Registration/Publication

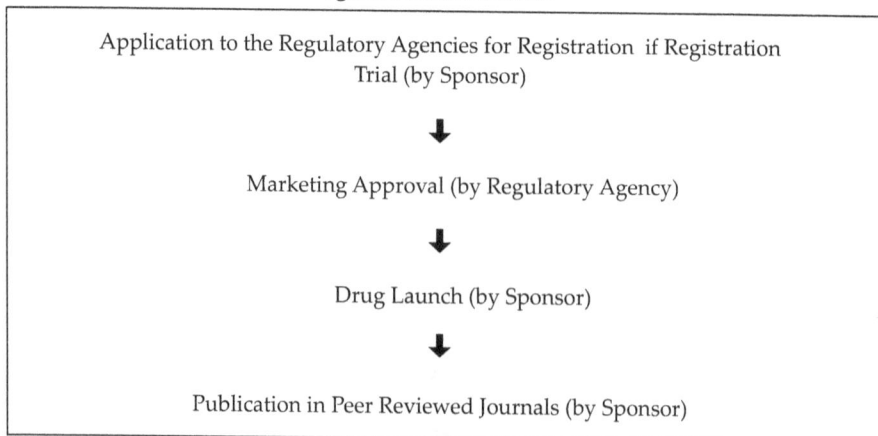

Application to the Regulatory Agencies for Registration if Registration Trial (by Sponsor)

↓

Marketing Approval (by Regulatory Agency)

↓

Drug Launch (by Sponsor)

↓

Publication in Peer Reviewed Journals (by Sponsor)

Location of Essential Documents Before, During and After Completion of a Clinical Trial

1. Location of Essential Documents Before the Clinical Phase of the Trial Commences:

Sl. No.	Section/ Subsection	Title of The Document	Located in Files of			
			IN	SP	CRO	IEC
1.	ICH-GCP (8.2.1)	Investigator's brochure	✓	✓	✓	✓
2.	ICH-GCP (8.2.2)	Signed protocol and amendments, if any, and sample case report form	✓	✓	✓	✓
3.	ICH-GCP (8.2.3)	Information given to trial subject - Informed consent form (including all applicable translations) - Any other written information - Advertisement for subject recruitment (if used)	✓ ✓ ✓	✓ ✓ ✗	✓ ✓ ✗	✓ ✓ ✓
4.	ICH-GCP (8.2.4)	Financial aspects of the trial	✓	✓	✓	✓
5.	ICH-GCP (8.2.5)	Insurance statement (where required)	✓	✓	✓	✓
6.	ICH-GCP (8.2.6)	Signed agreement between involved parties, *e.g.*: - Investigator/institution and Sponsor - Investigator/institution and CRO - Sponsor and CRO - Investigator/institution and Authority (ies) (where required)	 ✓ ✓ ✗ ✓	 ✓ ✓ ✓ ✓	 ✓ ✓ ✓ ✓	 ✓ ✓ ✗ ✓
7.	ICH-GCP (8.2.7)	Dated, documented approval/ favorable opinion of IRB/IEC of the following: - Protocol and any amendments - CRF (if applicable) - Informed consent form(s) - Any other written information to be provided to the subject(s) - Advertisement for subject recruitment (if used)	✓	✓	✓	✓

IN - Investigator; SP - Sponsor; IEC - Institutional Ethics Committee

Sl. No.	Section/ Subsection	Title of The Document	Located in Files of			
			IN	SP	CRO	IEC
		- Subject compensation (if any) - Any other documents given Approval/ favorable opinion	✓	✓	✓	✓
8.	ICH-GCP (8.2.8)	Institutional Review Board/ Independent ethics committee composition	✓	✓	✓	✓
9.	ICH-GCP (8.2.9)	Regulatory authority (ies) authorization/ approval/notification of protocol (where required)	✓	✓	✓	✓
10.	ICH-GCP (8.2.10)	Curriculum vitae and/or other relevant documents evidencing qualifications of Investigator(s) and Sub-Investigator(s)	✓	✓	✓	✓
11.	ICH-GCP (8.2.11)	Normal value(s) / range(s) for medical/laboratory / technical procedure(s) and/or test(s) included in the protocol	✓	✓	✓	✗
12.	ICH-GCP (8.2.12)	Medical / laboratory / technical procedures / Tests - Certification or - Accreditation or - Established quality control And/or external qualityAssessment or - Other validation (where Required)	✓	✓	✓	✗
13.	ICH-GCP (8.2.13)	Sample of label(s) attached to in-vestigational product container(s)	✗	✓	✓	✗
14.	ICH-GCP (8.2.14)	Instructions for handling of investigational product(s) and trial-related materials (if not included in protocol or Investigator's Brochure)	✓	✓	✓	✗
15.	ICH-GCP (8.2.15)	Shipping records for investigational product(s) and trial-related materials	✓	✓	✓	✗

IN - Investigator; SP - Sponsor; IEC - Institutional Ethics Committee

Sl. No.	Section/ Subsection	Title of The Document	Located in Files of			
			IN	SP	CRO	IEC
16.	ICH-GCP (8.2.16)	Certificate(s) of analysis of investigational product(s) shipped	✗	✓	✓	✗
17.	ICH-GCP (8.2.17)	Decoding procedures for blinded trials	✓	✓	✓	✗
18.	ICH-GCP (8.2.18)	Master randomization list	✓	✓	✓	✗
19.	ICH-GCP (8.2.19)	Pre-trial monitoring report	✗	✓	✓	✗
20.	ICH-GCP (8.2.20)	Trial initiation monitoring report	✓	✓	✓	✗

IN - Investigator; SP - Sponsor; IEC - Institutional Ethics Committee

2. Location of Essential Documents During the Clinical Conduct of a Trial:

Sl. No.	Section/ Subsection	Title of The Document	Located in Files of			
			IN	SP	CRO	IEC
1.	ICH-GCP (8.3.1)	Investigator's Brochure updates	✓	✓	✓	✓
2.	ICH-GCP (8.3.2)	Any revisions to: - Protocol/amendment(s) and CRF - Informed consent form - Any other written information provided to subjects - Advertisement for subject recruitment(if used)	✓	✓	✓	✓
3.	ICH-GCP (8.3.3)	Dated, documented approval/ favorable opinion of Institutional Review Board (IRB)/Independent ethics committee (IEC) of the following: - Protocol amendment(s) - Revision(s) of: - Informed consent form - Any other written information provided to subject - Advertisement for subject recruitment(if used) - Any other documents given approval / favorable opinion - Continuing review of trial	✓	✓	✓	✓
4.	ICH-GCP (8.3.4)	Regulatory authority(ies) authorizations / approvals / notifications where required for: - Protocol amendment(s) and other documents	✓	✓	✓	✓
5.	ICH-GCP (8.3.5)	Curriculum vitae for new investigator(s) and / or sub-investigator(s)	✓	✓	✓	✓
6.	ICH-GCP (8.3.6)	Updates to normal value(s)/ range(s) for medical/ laboratory/ technical procedure(s)/ test(s) included in the protocol	✓	✓	✓	✗

IN - Investigator; SP - Sponsor; IEC - Institutional Ethics Committee

Sl. No.	Section/ Subsection	Title of The Document	Located in Files of			
			IN	SP	CRO	IEC
7.	ICH-GCP (8.3.7)	Updates of Medical / laboratory / technical procedures / tests - Certification or - Accreditation or - Established quality control and / or external quality assessment or - Other validation (where required)	✓	✓	✓	✗
8.	ICH-GCP (8.3.8)	Documentation of investigational product(s) and trial-related materials shipment	✓	✓	✓	✗
9.	ICH-GCP (8.3.9)	Certificate(s) of analysis for new batches of investigational products	✗	✓	✓	✗
10.	ICH-GCP (8.3.10)	Monitoring visit reports	✗	✓	✓	✗
11.	ICH-GCP (8.3.11)	Relevant communications other than site visits - Letters - Meeting notes - Notes of telephone calls	✓	✓	✓	✗
12.	ICH-GCP (8.3.12)	Signed informed consent forms	✓	✗	✗	✗
13.	ICH-GCP (8.3.13)	Source documents	✓	✗	✗	✗
14.	ICH-GCP (8.3.14)	Signed, dated and completed case report forms (CRFs)	✓	✓	✓	✗
15.	ICH-GCP (8.3.15)	Documentation of CRF corrections	✓	✓	✓	✗
16.	ICH-GCP (8.3.16)	Notification by originating investigator to sponsor of serious adverse events and related reports	✓	✓	✓	✗
17.	ICH-GCP (8.3.17)	Notification by sponsor and/or investigator, where applicable, to regulatory authority(ies) and IRB(s)/ IEC(s) of unexpected serious adverse drug reactions and of other safety information	✓	✓	✓	✓

IN - Investigator; SP - Sponsor; IEC - Institutional Ethics Committee

Sl. No.	Section/ Subsection	Title of The Document	Located in Files of			
			IN	SP	CRO	IEC
18.	ICH-GCP (8.3.18)	Notification by sponsor to investigators of safety information	✓	✓	✓	✓
19.	ICH-GCP (8.3.19)	Interim or annual reports to IRB/ IEC and authority(ies)	✓	✓	✓	✓
20.	ICH-GCP (8.3.20)	Subject screening log	✓	✓	✓	✕
21.	ICH-GCP (8.3.21)	Subject identification code list	✓	✕	✕	✕
22.	ICH-GCP (8.3.22)	Subject enrolment log	✓	✕	✕	✕
23.	ICH-GCP (8.3.23)	Investigational product(s) accountability at the site	✓	✓	✓	✕
24.	ICH-GCP (8.3.24)	Signature sheet	✓	✓	✓	✕
25.	ICH-GCP (8.3.25)	Record of retained body fluids/ tissue samples (if any)	✓	✓	✓	✕

IN - Investigator; SP - Sponsor; IEC - Institutional Ethics Committee

3. Location of Essential Documents After Completion or Termination of the Trial:

Sl. No.	Section/ Subsection	Title of The Document	Located in Files of			
			IN	SP	CRO	IEC
1.	ICH-GCP (8.4.1)	Investigational product(s) accountability at site	✓	✓	✓	✗
2.	ICH-GCP (8.4.2)	Documentation of investigational product(s) destruction	✓	✓	✓	✗
3.	ICH-GCP (8.4.3)	Completed subject identification code list	✓	✗	✗	✗
4.	ICH-GCP (8.4.4)	Audit certificate (if required)	✗	✓	✓	✗
5.	ICH-GCP (8.4.5)	Final trial close-out monitoring report	✗	✓	✓	✗
6.	ICH-GCP (8.4.6)	Treatment allocation and decoding documentation	✗	✓	✓	✗
7.	ICH-GCP (8.4.7)	Final report by investigator/ institution to IRB/ IEC where required, and where applicable, to the regulatory authority (ies)	✓	✗	✗	✓
8.	ICH-GCP (8.4.8)	Clinical study report	✓	✓	✓	✗

IN - Investigator; SP - Sponsor; IEC - Institutional Ethics Committee

Critical Milestones of a Clinical Trial Project

Sl. No.	Milestone	Planned Date	Actual Date
1.	Preparation of Clinical Development Plan		
2.	Protocol Development		
3.	ICD Development		
4.	IB Development		
5.	CRF Development		
6.	Investigator Site Selection		
7.	IRB/IEC/EC Approval		
8.	Regulatory Submission		
9.	Database Set-up (Data Management)		
10.	Regulatory Approval		
11.	IP Import/ Procurement		
12.	Investigator's Training Meeting		
13.	First Patient Visit (FPV)		
14.	First Data to Database		
15.	Last Patient Enter Treatment (LPET)		
16.	Last Patient Visit (LPV)		
17.	Last Data to Database		
18.	Interim Data Lock		
19.	Final Data Lock		
20.	Site Closure		
21.	Clinical Study Report (CSR) Preparation		
22.	Trial Closure		
23.	Archival		

30

Overview of Regulatory Environment in USA, Australia, Europe, UK and India

Clinical Research Regulation in USA Food and Drug Administration (FDA)

Website: http://www.fda.gov

The U S. Food and Drug Administration is a scientific, regulatory, and public health agency. It is responsible for most food products (not meat and poultry), human and animal drugs, therapeutic agents of biological origin, medical devices, radiation-emitting products for consumer, medical, and occupational use, cosmetics, and animal feed.

The staff is composed of chemists, pharmacologists, physicians, microbiologists, veterinarians, pharmacists, lawyers and others. Agency scientists evaluate applications for new human drugs and biologics, complex medical devices, food and color additives, infant formulas, and animal drugs.

The FDA monitors the manufacture, import, transport, storage, and sale of about $1 trillion worth of products annually. The FDA visits more than 16,000 facilities a year, including manufacturing plants and clinical study sites.

Selected Regulations and Guidance for Drug Studies

The FDA publishes the Code of Federal Regulations (CFR). Stacked together, the fourteen or so books will reach 3 or 4 feet in height. Clinical trials related regulations are covered under CFR Title 21 Food and Drugs (which is revised frequently and published yearly) parts:

Part 11   Electronic records: electronic signatures
Part 50   Protection of human subjects
Part 54   Financial disclosure by clinical investigators
Part 56   Institutional Review Boards
Part 312   Investigational new drug application
Part 314   Applications for FDA approval to market a new drug

New Drug Approval Process at FDA

1.   Preclinical Testing
2.   Sponsor/ FDA Meetings (Pre-IND)
3.   Submission of IND to FDA
4.   Phase I Study
5.   Phase II Study
6.   Sponsor/ FDA Meetings (End of Phase II)
7.   Phase3 III Study
8.   Sponsor/ FDA Meetings (Pre-NDA)
9.   New Drug Application (NDA) Submission to FDA (for marketing approval)
10. FDA reviewers will either Approve the drug or find it Approvable, or Not Approvable
11. Permission for Marketing

12. Post Marketing Review

Investigational New Drug Application (IND)
After completing preclinical testing, a company files an IND with FDA to begin the testing of the drug in human. IND Application is the means through which sponsor (usually the manufacturer or potential marketer) obtains a legal status to call its new investigational molecule as new drug. The IND becomes effective if FDA does not disapprove it within 30 days.

Main components of an IND include:
- Description of the drug substance
- Chemistry, manufacturing and control information
- All known pre-clinical information
- Any previous human study reports
- Investigator's Brochure
- Clinical development plan
- Protocol and investigator list for the Phase I clinical trial

Each time a new study protocol or new study site is initiated or investigator is added to an ongoing protocol, the IND is amended. Protocol amendments also require an amendment to the IND.

New Drug Application (NDA)
An NDA is an application submitted to the FDA for permission to market a new drug product in the United States. Although the quantity of information and data submitted in NDA can vary significantly, the components of NDA are more uniform. NDA can consist of as many as 15 different sections:

- Index
- Summary
- Chemistry, Manufacturing, and Control
- Samples, Methods Validation Package, and Labeling
- Non-clinical Pharmacology and Toxicology
- Human Pharmacokinetics and Bioavailability
- Microbiology (for anti-microbial drugs only)
- Clinical Data
- Safety Update Report (typically submitted 120 days after the NDA's submission)
- Statistical Analysis
- Case Report Tabulations
- Case Report Forms
- Patent Information
- Patent Certification and Other Information

At the conclusion of FDA review of an NDA, there are three possible action letters that can be sent to the sponsor:
- Not Approvable Letter: It lists the deficiencies in the application and explains why the application cannot be approved.

- Approvable Letter: It signals that, ultimately, the drug can be approved and lists minor deficiencies that can be corrected, often involves labeling changes, and requests commitment to do post-approval studies.
- Approval Letter: It states that the drug is approved. It may follow an approvable letter, but can also be issued directly.

If the outcome is either Not Approvable Letter or Approvable Letter, FDA provides applicants an opportunity to meet with Agency officials and discuss the deficiencies. The purpose of the meeting is to discuss what further steps are necessary before the application can be approved.

Abbreviated New Drug Application (ANDA) and Abbreviated Antibiotic Drug Application (AADA)

An Abbreviated New Drug Application (ANDA) and Abbreviated Antibiotic Drug Application (AADA) is submitted to FDA's Center for Drug Evaluation and Research, Office of Generic Drugs for obtaining the approval to market a generic drug product.

Generic drug applications are termed "abbreviated" because these are not required to include preclinical (animal) and clinical (human) data to establish safety and effectiveness. Instead the applicant must scientifically demonstrate that their product is bioequivalent with the innovator drug.

SPECIAL CIRCUMSTANCES

Accelerated Development/Review

Accelerated development/review is a highly specialized mechanism for speeding the development of drugs that promise significant benefit over existing therapy for serious or life-threatening illnesses where no therapy exists. This process incorporates several novel elements aimed at making sure that rapid development and review is balanced by safeguards to protect both the patients and the integrity of the regulatory process.

The fundamental element of this process is that the manufacturers must continue testing after approval to demonstrate that the drug indeed provides therapeutic benefit to the patient. If not, the FDA can withdraw the product from the market more easily than usual.

Parallel Track

"Parallel track" policy is another mechanism in US to permit wider availability of experimental agents to patients with AIDS. Under this policy, patients with AIDS whose condition prevents them from participating in controlled clinical trials can receive investigational drugs that have shown promise in preliminary studies.

Clinical Hold Decision

When FDA does not believe, or cannot confirm, that the clinical study for the drug can be conducted without unreasonable risk to the subjects/patients, it places a "Clinical Hold" to the drug. If this occurs, the Center contacts the sponsor within the 30-day initial review period to stop the clinical trial. When a clinical hold is issued, a sponsor is required to address the issue that forms the basis of the hold before the order is removed.

Clinical Research Regulation in Australia- Therapeutic Goods Administration (TGA)

Website: http://www.tga.gov.au

The Australian drug regulatory agency is the Therapeutic Goods Administration (TGA). The TGA regulates the registration and marketing of all drugs and medical devices in Australia, as well as the conduct of clinical trials and compassionate use of unregistered drugs. Considering its relatively small size, the TGA is an internationally respected regulatory agency. Its rulings on approval (and rejection) of new drugs are keenly followed by most regional regulatory authorities, as well as those in Europe and North America.

The conduct of clinical trials in Australia comes under one of two schemes the CTX - Clinical Trial Exemption and the CTN - Clinical Trial Notification schemes. The CTX scheme requires a formal submission to be reviewed by TGA, and operates on a no objection basis. The CTX scheme requires a full submission including preclinical, pharmacology, safety, manufacturing and clinical data. This scheme also requires an Institutional Ethics Committee (IEC) approval.

The CTN, or Clinical Trial Notification scheme, on the other hand, is much simpler. Under this scheme, sponsors of clinical trials are required to obtain approval for their study from Human Research Ethics Committee (HREC) and an Institutional Ethics Committee (IEC), after which they simply notify the TGA of this approval and can commence their study.

Clinical Research Regulation in Europe-The European Agency for the Evaluation of Medicinal Products (EMEA)

Website: http://www.emea.europa.eu

The European Agency for the Evaluation of Medicinal Products (EMEA) is a decentralized body of the European Union. Its main responsibility is the protection and promotion of public and animal health, through the evaluation and supervision of medicines for human and veterinary use. The EMEA works as a network, bringing together the scientific resources of the Member States to ensure the highest level of evaluation and supervision of medicines in Europe. The Agency cooperates closely with international partners on a wide range of regulatory issues.

The EMEA is headed by the Executive Director and has a secretariat of staff members. A network of over 4000 European experts underpins the scientific work of the EMEA and its committees. The Agency's budget and work program are approved by the Management Board. The Board has two representatives from each Member State, from the European Parliament and from the European Commission.

The scientific opinions of the Agency are prepared by five committees responsible for medicines for human use (CPMP), for veterinary medicines (CVMP), for the designation of 'orphan' medicines, for rare diseases (COMP), for herbal medicinal products (HMPC) and the pediatric committee (PDCO). The CPMP and CVMP consist of two members nominated by each Member State. The COMP has one representative of each Member State, together with three representatives each of patient groups and of the EMEA.

Clinical Research Regulation in UK - Medicines & Healthcare Products Regulatory Agency (MHRA)

Website: http://www.mhra.gov.uk

The UK drug regulatory agency is the Medicines and Healthcare products Regulatory

Agency (MHRA) which replaced the Medical Devices Agency (MDA) and the Medicines Control Agency (MCA) in April 2003. The MHRA is the competent authority for medical devices and the Licensing Authority for pharmaceuticals advised by Committee on Safety of Medicines (CSM).

Key activities of MHRA are:
- Regulating medical devices
- Licensing of medicines before marketing and subsequent variations
- Regulation of clinical trials
- Operating adverse incident reporting system for medical devices
- Issuing safety warnings
- Responsibility for reporting, assessment and communications of defective medicines
- Monitoring of medicines and acting on safety concerns after marketing
- Evaluating medical devices to inform purchasing and encourage safe use
- Managing the General Practice Research Database (GPRD)
- Setting quality standards for drug substances through the "British Pharmacopoeia"
- Providing advice and guidance on medicines and medical devices

Clinical Research Regulation in India- Drug Controller General of India (DCGI)

Website: http://cdsco.nic.in

The Pharmaceutical business in India is governed by Drugs and Cosmetics Act 1940 (DCA), and the Drugs and Cosmetics Rules made there under. The legislation is enforced by the Central Government (Department of Chemicals and Fertilizers, Ministry of Chemicals and Petrochemicals) based at New Delhi. The office of Drug Controller General of India (DCGI) under Central Drug Standard Control Organization (CDSCO) has prime responsibility for regulating Clinical trials in India. Enforcement at the state level is done by the individual State Governments through their Food and Drug Administrations. Matters related to product approval and standards, clinical trials, introduction of new drugs, and import licenses for new drugs are handled by the DCGI. The approvals for setting up manufacturing facilities, and obtaining licenses to sell and stock drugs are provided by the State Governments.

In a nutshell, two Drug Organizations are functioning in India to exercise control over drugs:

1. Central Drug Standard Control Organization (CDSCO)
2. State Drug Control Organizations

Central Drug Standard Control Organization of the Government of India is headed by the Drugs Controller General (India). The prime responsibilities of this organization are:

- Controlling the quality of imported drugs;
- Coordinating the activities of the States and advising them on matters relating to the uniform administration of the Act in the country;
- Laying down rules and ancillary provisions of drug control and standards of drugs;
- Controlling the quality of drugs moving in inter-State commerce jointly with State Drug Control Organizations;
- Granting approval to "New Drugs" proposed to be imported or manufactured in the country;
- Controlling the quality of drugs which are exported from India;
- Arranging meetings of the two statutory bodies, namely the Drugs Technical Advisory

Board and the Drugs Consultative Committee and also processing all matters connected with their functioning.

Under the Drugs and Cosmetics Rules, the Drug Controller General (India) has been appointed as the Central License Approving Authority.

The Drugs Technical Advisory Board (DTAB) has technical experts and advises the Central and State Governments on all technical matters arising out of the enforcement of Drug Control. No rules can be made by the Central Government without consulting this Board.

The Drugs Consultative Committee has the Central and State Drug Control Officials as members, and its main function is to ensure that the Drug Control measures are enforced uniformly in all States.

Genetic Engineering Approval Committee (GEAC) is authority to approve rDNA pharmaceutical products. GEAC's role is to assess the bio-safety/environmental safety aspect of the biotechnological product.

Clinical Trials Guidelines in India

The guidelines that govern the conduct of clinical trials in India include:
- Revised Schedule Y (2005) of Drugs and Cosmetics Act, 1940
- Ethical Guidelines for Biomedical Research on Human Subjects, 2006
- Good Clinical Practices, 2001 (Indian GCP)

References
(in alphabetical order)

1. Association of the British Pharmaceutical Industry Amended May 1990. Guidelines for Medical Experiments in Non-Patient Human Volunteers. ABPI, London.

2. Drews J. Drug Discovery: A Historical Perspective. Science 2000; 287:1960-64.

3. Ethical Guidelines for Biomedical Research on Human Subjects, Indian Council of Medical Research, 2006.

4. Hillisch A, Hilgenfeld R. Modern Methods of Drug Discovery, Birkhauser, Germany, 2002.

5. Howard-Jones N. Human Experimentation in Historical and Ethical Perspectives. Soc Sci Med 1982; 16: 1429-48.

6. http://en.wikipedia.org/ [homepage on the Internet]: Wikipedia the Free Encyclopedia. Available from: http://en.wikipedia.org/wiki/Main_Page

7. http://www.cdsco.nic.in [homepage on the Internet]: New Delhi: Central Drugs Control Administration. Available from: http://www.cdsco.nic.in/index.html

8. http://www.emea.eu.int/ [homepage on the Internet]: European Medicines Agency.

9. http://www.fda.gov/ [homepage on the Internet]: U.S Food and Drug Administration.

10. http://www.tga.gov.au/ [homepage on the Internet]: Therapeutic Goods Administration, Australia.

11. ICH Guidelines for Good Clinical Practice, 1997. http://www.ich.org [homepage on the Internet]: E6 (R1): Switzerland: Good Clinical Practice: Consolidated Guidelines. Available from http://www.ich.org/LOB/media/MEDIA482.pdf

12. Julka P.K. Becoming a Successful Clinical Trial Investigator, 2nd Edition, DNA Press, Gurgaon, 2009.

13. Lakings DB. Making a Successful Transition from Drug Discovery to Drug Development, part 1. BioPharm 1995; 8(7): 20.

14. Mahajan BK. Methods in Biostatistics, 6th Edition, Jaypee Brothers, New Delhi, 2001.

15. Meinert C.L Clinical Trials: Design, Conduct and Analysis. Oxford University Press, New York, 1986.

16. Nielsen J.R. Handbook of Federal Drug Law. Lippincott, Williams and Wilkins, Philadelphia, 1992.

17. Pocock SJ. Clinical Trials: A Practical Approach. John Wiley and Sons, Chichester, 1983.

18. Schedule Y (Amended Version 2005). Available from: http://www.cdsco.nic.in/html/GCP1.html

19. Senn S. Cross-over Trials in Clinical Research. John Wiley and Sons, Chichester, 1993.

20. Siegel JP. Equivalence and Non-inferiority Trials. Am Heart J 2000; 139: 166-70.

21. Simon R. Optimal Two-stage Designs for Phase II Clinical Trials. Controlled Clinical Trials 1989; 10: 1-10.

22. Trials of War Criminals before the Nuremberg Military Tribunals under Control Council Law No. 10, Vol. 2, pp. 181-182. Washington, D.C.: U.S. Government Printing Office, 1949.

23. World Medical Association Declaration of Helsinki, Ethical Principles for Medical Research Involving Human Subjects, Adopted by the 18th WMA General Assembly Helsinki, Finland, June 1964 and its Subsequent Amendments.

www.ingramcontent.com/pod-product-compliance
Lightning Source LLC
Chambersburg PA
CBHW060444240326
41598CB00087B/3429